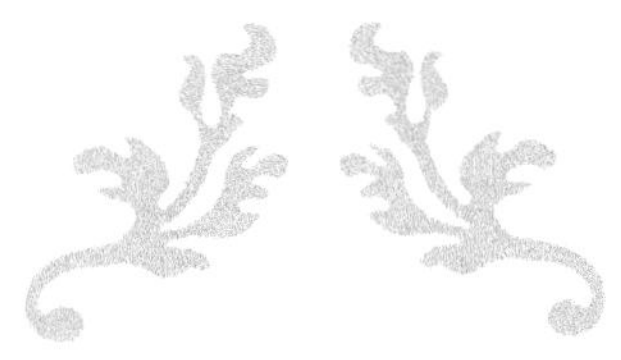

CAREGIVERS

SURVIVAL GUIDE

how to eliminate stress in 30 Minutes with

Chinese Medicine and other useful tools

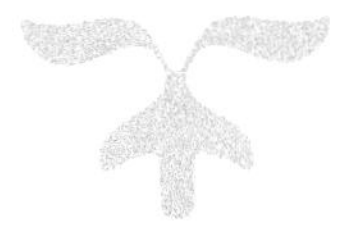

Kim Blaufuss, EAMP, Dipl Ac

ISBN: 978-1-7001-5967-0

Front cover image by Wolfgang Zwanzger/123rf.com
Book design by Kim Blaufuss/Kindle Create

Printed by Kindle Create, in the United States of America

First printing edition 2019

Best Acupuncture, LLC

PO Box 976

Woodland, WA 98674

www.best-acupuncture.com

Youtube @bestacupuncturellc

There are so many people I want to thank. I want to thank my sister and my mother. It was quite a life we led and without you, I never would have experienced our life. I miss you. My brother who taught me some hurts are just too much. My cousins Franz, David and Steve who remind me of a different past. My clients and friends who stayed by my side and through their support I was able to provide the support and care I wanted to give to my family. To my friends who read this book with me. Last and most importantly, to my husband who has supported me and been by my side through all of this and more. Love you.

-Kim

Contents

There are so many self-help books out there teaching you how to relax and unwind and find inner peace. You may wonder why this book would be any different. This book is geared to caregivers. It focuses on the stress caregivers feel and understands their time constraints. It doesn't require that you find a guru and spend years finding your inner sanctuary. In this book, I condense the ancient wisdom of Chinese medicine into a simple framework that you can use with no training and reap the benefits of 2,000 years of medicine.

It was during high school when my mother found she had Stage 3 breast cancer. My mom was the second person I knew to have breast cancer. At that time, I still believed that everyone lived forever. I didn't have a clue as to what Stage 3 meant.

My mother survived her initial encounter with cancer. She went through all the western treatments to overcome her disease. It worked. During her treatment, I remember her cancer sparked many great discussions with her friends over alternative treatments and fairy tale hopes. That was way back in the 1970s when China was opening up under Nixon, and words like

Acupuncture and Vegan were not even in our vocabulary. I knew one married couple in the WHOLE town who were vegans. What I really remembered about that couple was how sickly they looked.

Years later, my mother tested positive for Stage 3 Breast Cancer for the second time in her life. Only this time, she did something completely different and quite revolutionary. Based on those conversations she had so many years earlier, instead of chemo, radiation, and surgery, she decided to heal herself holistically with diet.

Wow!

Today I realize how brave she was to take that step. She would have received an insane amount of resistance and criticism. I was too young and naive to have such strong opinions about somebody else's health. I just knew the decision was hers. My father supported her. He supported her decision probably because he knew he didn't have a choice in the matter.

So, my mother and father packed their bags and headed out to Michio Kushi's Macrobiotic Institute in Massachusetts[1]. Today I am in awe of her raw

---

[1] Macrobiotics has been effective in womens' cancers

determination and courage to place her health and future in something as simple as diet. I am also experiencing a little hero envy. She not only got to meet the great Michio Kushi, but she was also able to work with him one-on-one and be trained by him.

That was my first introduction to the concept of disease as seen in the eyes of an Eastern practitioner. The body took on a new meaning. The personality, life, family, environment all had a role in her health. Food choices were made based on symptoms, as seen from an Eastern perspective.

And it worked! A few years later, my mother went back to her Western doctor. He expressed disbelief she was still alive. He had thought she had passed away. At that time, it was believed everyone died who didn't treat Stage 3 Breast Cancer with Western medicine. Of course, even with treatment, she could have passed.

She hadn't passed away. In fact, she was in complete remission. The cancer was gone. My mother

---

because the cancer is fat-based. Macrobiotics being an organic, detoxing, and weight reducing eating program is believed to be effective on fat based cancers.

survived her cancer and lived the remaining decades of her life cancer-free passing away at 82.

That was the start. It was a fantastic introduction to Eastern medical thought. Instead of the Western therapeutic approach of full-scale war with a winner takes all mentality, Macrobiotics showed compassion and left the body intact. She got stronger and healthier. The diminishment of the disease was the opening of life for her.

Very different from watching Western cancer treatment where the elimination of the disease risked the elimination of the individual. The hope was that the individual was still alive if they ever got the disease under control.

From that point on, I had wanted to be a Chinese Medical practitioner. It wasn't until much later in life that I was able to get up the courage to leave my corporate job and go back to school to study Chinese Medicine.

It was always the right decision. Life changes when you are doing something you love. It becomes easy and automatic. There were ups and downs, but the medicine satiated my need for constant growth, and the field is just so big. With growth came new learnings and new experiences.

I was able to incorporate Chinese Medicine, with the Five Element theory, into every aspect of my life. The more I learned about Chinese Medicine, the more flexible the medicine became. Its simplicity began to stick out. I started to learn to use it in very complicated situations with little or no effort. Unlike Western medicine, every time I used Chinese Medicine to address an issue, the life didn't diminish, it became more significant.

And that's where this book fits in your overall stress-free wellness plan. This is geared towards the individual who has enough on their plate as it is. Suddenly being confronted with significant stressors caregivers receive from multiple different directions can be overwhelming. Finding time to drive 30 minutes or more to talk to someone usually doesn't fit into our life when we are working 8-12 hours a day with a 45-minute commute each way. Just getting home gives us barely enough time to gobble down some crappy food and go to bed so we can do it all over again tomorrow.

So, here is your chance to introduce yourself to Eastern medical thought and find an effective way to get a quick, short-term stress fix. You can use it anywhere. You'll get to learn more about yourself, and you will enhance your life.

Introduction

It didn't really start with me. It started with my clients. It began with them coming in and asking me to treat things with needles and herbs that years of Western medicine or Western Counseling therapy hadn't been able to dent. These requests made me nervous. Like most United States and Chinese students of Chinese Medicine, I was trained in Traditional Chinese Medicine, as taught under Mao's China.

Under Mao, Traditional Chinese Medicine looked at all that was Chinese Medicine and tried to skinny the medicine down to just the physical manifestation of the disease. The spiritual, emotional, and mental aspects of Classical Chinese medicine were considered superstition and unscientific. Thus, Traditional Chinese Medicine became a reduction in Classical Chinese Medicine.

In Classical Chinese medical thought, the physical manifestation of the disease is the last expression. The disease starts much earlier in a person. I suppose Western medicine kind of realizes that. Yet, Western medicine has no science to support that kind of thinking. Chinese medicine did and does.

The disease starts back in the Dao with your karma. How your spirit incorporates your karma will spill over to your emotions. Your emotions affect your mental attitude and self-talk. When these aspects are out of balance, the potential for any disease exists. Time and patience allow an illness to manifest.

Traditional Chinese Medicine focuses on the last step. When I left school, I focused on the final expression of illness and avoided everything else. I had seen too many woo-woo practitioners that talked about peace, love, and karmic unity and couldn't deliver.

When a client came in and asked me to focus on the mental, emotional, and spiritual; I kind of balked at the notion. I didn't want to be one of those woo-woo guys.

Being narrow-minded comes in all shapes and forms, and I wasn't even sure I could work on the mental, emotional, and spiritual. It wasn't that Traditional Chinese Medicine students were not taught how to treat the mental, emotional, and spiritual in school. We were given the correct tools, just not how to look at the problem from that perspective.

I took a deep breath, thought about the problem, my toolset, and found a beacon of light showing me a direction. I grabbed it. I remember being very clear with the patient. I told him I didn't know what I was doing, but if there was anything to the theory, what I was doing might work. We were off.

About two months later, the patient, who had suffered decades of rage against his father, got up from the table, stared at me, and said, "It's gone. The rage is gone."

Oh my gosh, halleluiah, it was like an angel came down and helped guide my hand and my thoughts. It turned out to be just the right guidance to help push him back into balance.

That was the start. I realized there was so much more to Chinese Medicine then I was practicing.

Years later, I was going to be able to open my mind further. I found another side of Chinese Medicine. When I became a caregiver, Chinese Medicine helped me through one of the most stressful times of my life.

It started as a storm far offshore with small waves and a slight wind that, over the next three years, was going to grow into a hurricane pummeling us with gale-force winds. Crushing us under the oppressive, fierce weight of the tidal waves.

I think what made this especially significant is the generation I come from. I could be either the end of the baby boomers or the beginning of Generation X. Either way, we are a generation still working, and our kids are grown. We are young enough, our parents are still alive. The financial crises of the last two decades have wiped out the financial stability of our parents and our kids and shaken our own financial security. We are the first generation that is getting squeezed from both ends.

Our kids or grandkids are moving in with us. Our parents are moving in with us or requiring our time as a caregiver. Our spouse may be suffering from health issues. And it's much more complicated. There are all sorts of legal issues that didn't exist when we were raising a family. There are end of life legal issues that need to be addressed. What could have been handled effectively with a simple phone call 20 years ago, takes days and research, and repeated follow-ups to try and make the best decision.

I still remember the frustration when I was trying to figure out the insurance supplement for my mom and how much effort that took. I was talking with a retired senior citizen the other night. She stated she worked in and retired from the insurance industry. She knows how to read an insurance policy. She had thought she purchased a supplemental with acupuncture coverage. When she went to use the plan, she found the plan didn't cover acupuncture. This example highlights the lack of transparency in issues facing caregivers.

The other thing I didn't realize is your life doesn't take a back seat as a caregiver. Your life ceases to exist. You can't just check out, especially if the person you are caregiving for is starting to experience health issues, and the problems impair their ability to function.

My husband and I stopped doing everything we use to do. No date nights, no fun in the sun, no vacations. We were continually babysitting. At the end of it, we were strong, but we were strangers to each other. How we came back from that abyss is a different story. This story is about the tools we used to survive this period of our life.

The one thing that made caregiving especially tough is my "generation" is getting up in years. Our own health is becoming a concern. In fact, my husband and I had just started taking our health seriously. We had gone on a diet, focused on exercise, and started keeping current with our medical check-ups. We were beginning to relax into this time of our life. According to Chinese Medicine, this should be the harvest of our life. This is the time when we get to enjoy the fruits of our labor. And we were.

I've seen many different flavors of caregiving and the toll it takes on the caregiver. I believe my role was tough, but I've seen tougher.

I have one client whose husband suffers Alzheimer's. He still lives at home. He needs constant care. Where her situation becomes so painful is when she comes in. I can see their past. I can see they were best friends. I can see, they, like my husband and I did everything together. They were each other's foundation and each other's home.

Watching her and the level of stress, grief, remorse she experiences daily as she tries to come to grip with living her life alone really tears me apart.

I was naive when my husband talked about taking care of my family members. I knew it was likely going to happen. I blew off the conversation because it was too stressful to think about. I couldn't begin to guess how to prepare for such an event. Even if I tried to do something about it, all the legal issues and other issues have gotten so complicated.

Then it happens. You are a caregiver. I had thought the most complicated part would be the logistics of caregiving. Yet, when you are in it, the emotions surface, which are confusing and dismaying. You are caregiving for people you love and care about. However, having to be their caregiver 24x7 starts to bring up feelings of resentment, anger, hostility, grief. Having to incorporate these feelings into everything else happening is really overwhelming and confusing. How could you have these emotions for someone who you love so deeply? How can grief be coupled with relief when they are gone? The feelings were another aspect of being a caregiver I was not prepared for.

All these stressors, coupled with the stressors of everyday living and working and come together to form the essence of being a caregiver today. Caregiving starts out easy because you have a lot of vitality at the start of the process. But time is like water slowly wearing away the rock. As time flows by, you find yourself with less and less vitality. Stress starts to consume more time.

Self-care really becomes a novel concept because there just isn't any time. My husband and I struggled with this concept throughout our caregiving. I was working fulltime and felt terrible that he had to spend his days taking care of my mom. So, I would come home and try and assume that responsibility. That meant I had absolutely ZERO time to myself. It was tough for my recently retired husband as the house was his own time. He had absolutely ZERO private time anymore.

It became a process of trying to find quick ways to decompress while still staying close to the caregiving situation. That meant I couldn't take a couple of hours to drive to a weekly self-help meeting or any other self-care thing that was going to take me away and take a few hours. I had to find ways to decompress that could work quickly and without shirking my life responsibilities. I had to find a way to incorporate my self-care into my caregiving with my husband.

Thankfully, both my husband and I are still standing. Part of thanks comes from the process of writing this book. With insights from Chinese Medicine, the book was able to give us a moment to sit in the eye of the storm as we waited for it to pass. I found that Chinese Medicine had already taught me how to decompress quickly using my current environment. I just had to listen.

Come with me as I take you on a journey into the world of caregiving and Chinese Medicine. Learn more about what caregiving is and who caregiving impacts. Get introduced to Chinese Medicine with simple, easy to understand explanations. Get charts that will allow you to better understand Chinese Medicine and maybe better understand yourself. Learn how you can incorporate Chinese Medicine into your life to help weather the tidal waves of caregiving.

Chinese Medicine was able to give me a break when I had no time. Chinese Medicine could rebalance my emotional state when I felt like I was alone. Chinese Medicine gave me resolution and self-forgiveness when the emotions were overwhelming. I don't know who I would be or if I would have made it without Chinese Medicine.

PART 1: Who are Caregivers and what do we do?

I didn't really know the true meaning of altruism until now.

-Kim

Definition

So, we're all in here?

-Kim

The definition has expanded over the last 20 years. Depending on the survey, caregivers include parents taking care of children with disabilities, or grandparents assuming the role of parent to grandchildren, and taking care of an ailing spouse.

The definition has been expanding to include lifestyle factors that help better understand the demographics of caregivers. The definition incorporates financial implications, length of time in a caregiver role, hours a week spent caregiving, working status, educational status, age of the caregiver, and on and on and on.

When you look at all this data, you start to realize that caregivers are everyone, including you and me. Caregivers touch all walks of life. Their numbers are increasing.

The first thing about caregiving is caregiving doesn't happen slowly. You don't get to prepare for the experience. You don't get four years to go to Caregiving College. Usually, one day you wake-up and there you are. The experience is more a baptism by fire. Even if you think you prepared for the day, the true magnitude of the experience waits until you are so far in you can no longer back out and run.

The biggest challenge is the caregiving learnings. The learnings and lessons come in fast. You finish one, and a new one pops up before the dust settles on the old experience. You might find each item in caregiving is a whole new field taking extensive research. A caregiving item may be finding outside services to help with daily activities such as food shopping, people to check on them, or finding events for socializing. You might have to learn about insurance and insurance supplementals. For our aging population and especially for the one you love, you may end up in the role of a healthcare advocate learning to talk and plan with doctors and medical professionals. You might find yourself helping or managing the legal aspects of end of life or making the end of life decisions.

It is not just learning how to do the process of aging, the learnings are also emotional. In older adults and adults with disabilities, as their situation deteriorates, you may find their personality takes on a more prominent and more significant role in the household. You may be walking a strange line of a loved adult trying to maintain their independence and lifestyle. They are unaware they are experiencing emotional or physical changes.

Having to walk a tight rope leaves little time to grieve over this loss of the person you love. Unresolved grief can add a level of confusion to the whole process increasing the level of stress. You may find you don't have time to put down the caregiving role. You don't have time to process through your own personal loss. The caregiving process keeps going on and on. It seems to pick up steam as time progresses... almost like a boulder rolling downhill. The stone will only stop when it decides to stop. The best you can do is try to stay ahead of it.

There are some consistencies expressed by caregivers. The most commonly expressed unmet need is time for their own life. That could be finding time for themselves, managing emotional or physical stress, or finding time for their family and friends.

There is a "Level of Burden Index[2]," which helps identify the level of participation which you, as the caregiver, have assumed. I bring up the "Level of Burden Index" because the index can help you identify or justify your internal turbulence.

When you can't see the forest through the trees, it is hard to understand where you are in the big picture. It can become difficult to find direction or be aware you need to start walking.

When I look at the data on caregivers in more depth, some trends emerge. Overall, the age group of caregivers has been increasing. From 2004 to 2009, the average age of the caregiver increased from 46.4 to

---

[2] National Alliance for Caregiving, & AARP. (1997). *Family Caregiving in the Us Findings on a National Survey. Family Caregiving in the US Findings on a National Survey.* National Alliance for Caregiving and American Association of Retired Persons. Retrieved from https://assets.aarp.org/rgcenter/il/caregiving_97.pdf

49.2. But don't count out the younger millennials. The research that really shocked me was that 1 in 6 millennials[3] was in a caregiver role raising children with physical and emotional issues.

During the same five-year period, there has been an increase in unpaid caregivers[4], and a decrease is paid caregivers[5]. The most commonly identified reason for the decline in paid caregiver assistance was affordability.

---

[3] National Alliance for Caregiving, & American Association of Retired Persons. (2009). *Caregiving in the Us 2009. Caregiving in the US 2009*. National Alliance for Caregiving and AARP. Retrieved from https://www.caregiving.org/data/Caregiving_in_the_US _2009_full_report.pdf

[4] Youth Against Alzheimer's, & USC Suzanne Dworak-Peck. (2017). *Millennials and Dementia Caregiving in the United States. Millennials and Dementia Caregiving in the United States.* Youth Against Alzheimer's and USC Suzanne Dworak-Peck. Retrieved from https://www.usagainstalzheimers.org/sites/default/fil es/Dementia Caregiver Report_Final.pdf

[5] National Alliance for Caregiving, & American Association of Retired Persons. (2009). *Caregiving in the Us 2009. Caregiving in the US 2009*. National Alliance for Caregiving and AARP. Retrieved from https://www.caregiving.org/data/Caregiving_in_the_US _2009_full_report.pdf

Caregiving has a broad definition and includes all manner of care for related and unrelated individuals who are unable to take care of themselves. As a caregiver, you take on many more roles and responsibilities, and the roles and responsibilities tend to increase rather than decrease over time. Inevitably over time, the most significant unmet needs of the caregiver have been finding time to themselves and dealing with stress.

Why is it different

The amount of strength it takes to be a caregiver is nothing compared to the amount of strength it takes to say goodbye.

-Kim

For many, being a caregiver is going to be your most challenging experience. Most are not trained to be a caregiver. It just happens. Based on prior life experiences, you tumble through caregiving like being tossed into river rapids and having to make it to shore.

Besides an increasing average age for caregivers, there is one additional change happening in caregiving. Caregivers may be caring for more than one generation like grandchildren, children, a spouse, or parents.

Caregiving adults are at a time in life when most of the trauma and struggle of life has settled down. They are established in jobs, communities, and friendships. All the work they did in their 20's, 30's, and 40's laid a foundation that is starting to pay-off. They are finally beginning to reap what has been sown.

And just in time, too, because this is also the time when health starts to take center stage. All the vitality which, in youth, kept disease at bay is less available with aging. As the caregivers age, most of them won't have the energy that allowed them to stay up all night with a sick child and go to work the next day. All the abuse which your body sustained in your earlier years is starting to catch up to us.

Long-term health concerns like obesity, diabetes, high blood pressure, and high cholesterol start to appear, requiring decisions about managing health. For many, caregiving is going to be a challenge because it is happening when the caregiver is much older.

Your energy was used to manage a growing family, advance careers, obtain an education, and things related to achieving our life's goals. Now, age means the need to rest and take things a bit slower. Now what is sought after is less drama, less responsibility at work, more free time, and more fun.

What It Looks Like

I had no idea...

-Kim

Two significant drivers make caregiving unique. First, this is the first generation that may be asked to be a caregiver for multiple generations: grandchildren, children, spouse, friends, or parents. You have the genuine possibility of being the caregiver to more than one generation, and the data is also showing that the populations needing caregivers are expanding at an aggressive rate.

Grandparents taking care of grandchildren increased 76% between 1970 and 1997.[1] In 2011-2012, it was estimated that an average of 39.6 million civilians were unpaid caregivers[2]. In 2015, the count had increased to 43.9 million civilians[3], an increase of 11% over three years.

The diseases which require some managed care, such as Alzheimer's [4][5], are increasing and targeting younger generations. In 2013, it was estimated that 5.4 million people have Alzheimer's disease. By 2050, it is predicted to increase to 13.8 million.

You can become a caregiver at any time, but the data is showing it is more likely to happen in your 50's and 60's [6]. Today, it is a different generation experiencing a squeeze from both ends. The financial chaos of the preceding 20 years has wiped out savings accounts and sabotaged employment opportunities making financial stress a key reason for caregivers to multiple generations.

Senior parents, unable to take care of themselves and without financial opportunities, end up relying on their children to help them through the end of their life. In just the same way, children, their new family, or their children's children unable to provide in today's economy turn towards their parents for help. This generation's youth, young adults, and young parents moving in with family is an expanding phenomenon.

When I grew up, the job market was strong enough to maintain me outside of the family, and education was super affordable. I had to work hard to establish myself. But it was achievable.

The generation before me is truly the last generation that had the opportunity to retire fully. Yet, retirement for them is not guaranteed. Pummeled by the economic chaos of the previous couple of decades, many aging adults lost everything they had saved through one calamity after another. Fewer of this older generation can experience retirement. Physically capable parents may find themselves needing to move in with their children.

My long-term financial plan, when I grew up, did not include taking care of my parents. I grew up at a time where company loyalty, retirements from work, social security, and savings were established and could take care of our seniors in their later life. Through cost-cutting, corporate downsizing, lost pensions, corporate take-overs, technology advances, and globalization, this security has disappeared. When I found myself in the position of taking care of my elder parent, the expense of eldercare had not been factored into my financial planning.

Financial Strain

I'd like to say it's not about money, but sometimes it is...

-Kim

The actual out-of-pocket financial costs of caregiving turned out to be more then I was expecting. I thought the overall impact of adding someone to my established household would be insignificant. I didn't consider the additional costs when my husband and I started our role of caregiving for my elderly mother.

Within the first year, our financial status began to show strain. We were not monitoring the added costs of caregiving because we didn't think it was substantial.

Yet, by the end of the first year, we had cut back all our miscellaneous expenditures including eating out, vacations, toys. We started laying out our budget to try and get a handle on why our expenditures seemed so out of control!

Even though you think adding one more person will not be a significant increase, for caregiving families, the increase in household expenses can be as much as 20% of their annual income or more.[6] It is estimated to be slightly more costly to be a caregiver for an adult than a child.[7] The actual estimated dollar amount spent annually is between $7K and $12K for basic life expenses.[8]

Some of the more common additional expenses include ADA doorways, ADA compliant bathrooms to include toilets, roll-in showers, appropriate counter heights, etc. Other things may be hallways that

[6] AARP Research, Rainville, C., Skufa, L., & Mehegan, L. (2016). *Family Caregivers Cost Survey: What They Spend and What They Sacrifice. Family Caregivers Cost Survey: What They Spend and What They Sacrifice.* AARP. Retrieved from https://www.aarp.org/research/topics/care/info-2016/family-caregivers-cost-survey.html

[7] AARP Research, Rainville, C., Skufa, L., & Mehegan, L. (2016). *Family Caregivers Cost Survey: What They Spend and What They Sacrifice. Family Caregivers Cost Survey: What They Spend and What They Sacrifice.* AARP. Retrieved from https://www.aarp.org/research/topics/care/info-2016/family-caregivers-cost-survey.html

[8] AARP Research, Rainville, C., Skufa, L., & Mehegan, L. (2016). *Family Caregivers Cost Survey: What They Spend and What They Sacrifice. Family Caregivers Cost Survey: What They Spend and What They Sacrifice.* AARP. Retrieved from https://www.aarp.org/research/topics/care/info-2016/family-caregivers-cost-survey.html

accommodate wheelchairs, ADA accessible bedrooms and doorways, and on and on. Lighting and ramps are additional features. Safety technology may be needed. You may need a van capable of transporting them to appointments or with the ability for a wheelchair bound person to drive the vehicle. Requirements will vary based on individual needs.

Financial costs can include medical expenses which can be insurance costs, paid caregiver costs, or facility costs. Other costs that may not be covered by insurance can increase as level of care needed increases.

Moving an adult to a new location incurs added costs. If you are moving them out of the house they lived in for 30 years, the actual packing and moving can take months. Some of the costs can be costs for travel, time off work, storage costs, moving boxes, packing material, moving vans, auction costs, legal costs, legal costs to ramp down the home, insurance, taxes and a host of other costs.

Caregivers also rely more on technology to help with monitoring the adult. Technology has equipment costs, installation costs, monitoring fees and learning curves.

These are just a few of the costs that you may face and can make caregiving a little costly.

Technology

The one thing I learned is that my ability to survive aging is going to be predicated on technology.

-Kim

Technology is such a massive boon to caregivers today. Techonology can reduce stress by giving much better control over remote caregiving. With technology, you know what is going on, can easily monitor and talk to the person, and can ensure they are in a safe place. Advances are going on in technology that will ensure I will be able to live unassisted for a much longer time.

Even though technology gives a substantial boost to the growing caregiver industry, the technology focus is really to allow seniors more independence and freedom in a safe environment. Beware, even though technology allows for much more freedom, technology does not replace the human connection people need to survive.

How do you focus on keeping your loved ones safe while still allowing them some form of independence? Technology was the tool that I used to help me navigate some of the safety issues with caregiving.

I got lucky with Alexa. Amazon had put a lot of effort into this tool as Amazon raced to develop home artificial intelligence. The technology had some great features. The ability to drop-in and talk to the senior at any time is a great feature. The drop-in feature could be used with Alexa's ability to video conference so they could see you, and you could see them. That wasn't the only way I used Alexa, I asked Alexa to deliver reminders. These reminders would go off at a chosen time and helped remind my parent to take medications, appointments, or whatever other reminders are needed. Your loved one can order Uber or call a family member all by talking to Alexa.

Some people like Google's apps. I just found that, overall, their apps were not as robust or customer-centric. That doesn't mean you can't use them. You can. The biggest detractor for me was a higher failure rate with Google software.

Camera technology can monitor movement, home temperature, air quality. Doorbells, like the Ring, can watch who comes to the door. They allow you to talk over the intercom with the person at the door. I purchased and tested out four different camera systems to identify the system right for me. The four systems we tested were the hard-wired Ring system, Canary, Swann wired system, and Yi cameras. Everyone is going to have different criteria, and my criteria and why I decided on one camera over another is documented under the section "Emotions: Fear."

Switches allow lights and other electrical equipment to be programmed remotely to come on and off. We tried switches that were on timers, and those work well. I just felt they were dated. I had wanted something that I had more control over when I wasn't there. I wanted to be able to change the program or turn on and off lights and equipment when I wanted. I wanted to be able to do this all remotely. I only had to check out one switch, and that was the Wemo. The Wemo worked as advertised and, not only could you use it for equipment that plugs into a wall socket, you could use it to add automation to light switches. So, instead of having to find the wall switch, I could use Wemo, hook up to Alexa, walk into the room, and say, "Alexa, turn on bedroom light." Or lay in bed and say, "Alex, turn off bedroom light." Wemo connects wirelessly to your internet. I downloaded the app. I did some minimal scheduling and was in business.

On some lights, I wanted to have them come on if they sense movement. All the motion sensing wall light switches worked as advertised. You can buy them at Home Depot, Lowes, Ace, True Value, or any other building supply store. We just had to replace the existing wall light switch with a motion-sensing light switch from one of these stores. For me, motion sensors were a good option for bathrooms and hallways. The lights automatically turn on when someone walks into the area. After a period of no movement, the switch automatically turns off the lights.

Ecobee or Nest allows you to monitor, change, and maintain the air and heating unit in the home remotely. My husband found you had to read through all the information on each system to determine which one really works best for you. We went with the Ecobee. Not only can you schedule and manage the temperature, but Ecobee will also keep you up to date with your maintenance schedule. You can add more temperature sensors to the Ecobee. Although I use multiple sensors and they work, how Ecobee incorporates the data and determines the average temperature is a little bit....meh...

Smartphones can bring all this together. My husband and I use smartphones. The apps are usually free, there is more programming for smartphones, and smartphones are taking more market share. Smartphones are a more extensive choice when companies expand their technology. The best thing about the smartphone is it can control all the technology. You can be anywhere in the United States and hook up to the internet to review all your technology, drop-in on your senior, manage their furnace, etc., etc. Yet, the most essential thing, smartphones have GPS locating and allowing you to monitor and track where your adult is. On smartphones, the google location on the maps application is free and usually works.

The only problem with locating your senior is when the person doesn't keep their phone with them. I know! Who doesn't keep their phone with them? For most of us, it has become a new appendage. But, for seniors? They didn't grow up with these phones and don't see the use of them. For the person who isn't good about keeping their phone on them, some of the new GPS locating technology can help.

There are some different GPS locating tags that may help here. These are small square devices that are about the size of a two-inch square. I know, crazy. You use these things to track where your drone landed when you have accidentally flown it out of range.

They have a lot more uses than just keeping track of things. You can drop this square device into a purse, wallet, onto a vehicle, or whatever it is you think will be with them when they leave the house. You need to review the different trackers and make sure it has what you need. I wanted a long battery life, like a few months. You don't want to have to keep pulling out the tracker to recharge it. The more independent seniors might not appreciate it, figure out what the device is, and conveniently leave the device at home when they leave. Some of the trackers have satellite, which allows for remote management of location like Google locate. Others have a limited range of a couple miles. That can be o.k. if you are only worried about when they go out for a walk. Others have a short range of a few hundred feet and are not useful for monitoring a person's location.

Then there are the smartwatches with phone numbers and GPS. They allow the senior to wear a watch and call a few phone numbers. The watches are marketed to parents for their children and are network limited. Contact your cell phone carrier for options.

The technology is growing and expanding, with Artificial Intelligence becoming more and more ingrained in the market. The features available today are going to expand and change tomorrow. Yet, this is the list of things I used at the forefront of the industry.

Changes to Your Personal Life

It just happens and I didn't even notice until I was so deep into caregiving. -Kim

Loss of independence for seniors and disabled persons has different definitions. Here is a four-stage method of defining loss of independence. Note that safety concerns can arise during any of these stages.

1. The first stage is the adult who can live on their own and is physically independent.

2. The second stage is the adult who is independent inside the home but may need help outside the home. This can include tasks like help getting to appointments, finding professionals such as hairdressers or attorneys, shopping, or driving.

3. The third stage is when the adult needs help with daily activities both inside and outside the house. These can be tasks such as getting assistance with dressing, making meals, help with showers, or the toilet. With the rapid change in technology, they may need help working with televisions, video players, phones.

4. The fourth stage is the adult who is bedridden throughout the day. At this level, the adult does not need to be mentally incapacitated. I knew a practicing alcoholic who was intellectually coherent. His body had just given out. At this level, all physical

tasks need assistance such as bathing, toilet, eating, changing clothes, bedsheets.

As a caregiver, progressing through each of these levels takes more and more of your personal time. At each level, there will be emotionally trying tasks you will have to complete. At stage two, the most challenging task is having to take away the car keys. For most aging adults removing car keys is a pivotal blow to their independence and a critical reminder of their mortality. For some adults, there is a fear associated with aging, which includes fear of abandonment, fear of loss of freedom, fear of losing family, and familiar surroundings.

Probably the most common fear through all of it is, "How will I manage"? Having to give up the car keys is the first real marker things are happening. They are aging, and the reality of aging is now at their door.

For the caregiver, tasks like having to take away the car keys can be a thankless task and sometimes takes a lot of creativity to weather the storm. I have a friend who took her mom to the DMV to renew her mom's license. My friend stood behind her mom while her mom took the eye exam. Throughout the eye exam, my friend signaled to the tester to fail her mother. It was a small town, and the examiner knew my friend. The examiner failed her mother, and everyone went home happy except her mom. The moral of the story? Her mom didn't focus her frustrations and fear on her children. She focused her fear on the system.

Taking away the car keys may be a thankless task, but in the second stage, you are now responsible for coordinating and managing all their appointments. You may already be working through the status of their bills, financials, legal obligations. You are starting to manage their life. You are responsible for making appointments, as well as transporting them to their appointments and so on. This is an excellent time to create a health history binder to take with you to all appointments.

Managing a life that isn't yours, and figuring out what needs to be done isn't easy. Missing a task that needs to be done can be costly, either emotionally or financially. Sometimes stepping in to manage someone else's life is more like a game of clue and can get even messier if more than one hand is stirring the pot.

When you are caregiving for a senior in stage two, you are starting to lose your social life. Your free time is being allocated to the person who needs your care - your second life. And you may begin to experience some financial implications draining your finances. Thus, even if you wanted a social life, you don't have the extra money to have a social life.

Moving to the next stage, stage three is where things can get complicated. Here the adult can start to lose all independence. Dementia or Alzheimer's can be a real concern. Speech may be affected making it difficult for anyone, other than a close family member, to understand and communicate. The adult can start to panic when their caregiver is out of sight, making them combative. They may not be bedridden, but they are taking 24x7 care, and the caregiver has wholly lost their life.

If the caregiver is working, it can become a struggle to juggle caregiving with work. You never know what is going to happen. One morning they might fall out of bed, requiring an emergency visit to the hospital. Another morning they might accidentally knock their breakfast onto the bed or floor. You might not be able to get their daily clothes on.

Anything can happen at level three. You are doing more than just managing their life, you are their life. Just because you are their life doesn't mean you can plan their life. They still control all the emotional responses that drive their actions. Even though you are their life, someone else is driving the car.

You already lost your social life at level two. At level three is where your friends can go incognito. Caregiving is a trying task. Caring for the elderly is confusing, and the adult may be loved but cannot participate in social gatherings even though they want to participate. Due to aging or personality, the adult may be difficult to be around.

Our current lifestyles compound this issue. We are very much a "Do It Yourself" culture, which precludes working together. Our family units are dispersed across the continent. Which means we don't have family nearby to help. We've also read so many books about boundaries and not dealing with unacceptable or inconvenient behavior that we are intolerant. All these things have almost turned off our compassion meter.

If you are a caregiver, when you are through your caregiving, you'll have already experienced this next part. For those of you who haven't been through a caregiving role, think how it must be for the caregiver. If it is so uncomfortable for you that you don't want to be around for a half-hour, realize the caregiver is dealing with this 24x7 with absolutely no breaks.

My advice to you, if there is one thing you can do for a caregiver, it is to reach out to them. Stop by, call, or take a minute and take over the responsibility of caregiving, for even an hour, to allow them to have a moment to themselves. Just this small act of kindness can give them enough of a break to have the strength to carry on.

I never really thought about it, but my sister's fiancé had melanoma. The cancer had progressed and was terminal. He went through treatments and did the macrobiotic diet. Every time things started turning around for him, another shoe would drop. He would get another cancer. A new treatment would come in, and things would look good, and then it would be something else.

He ran out of options. The Western Medical community couldn't treat him anymore. Today you would be surprised at where the doctor's stopped treating my sister's fiancé. He was still standing and moving around and could have a life for a short time. More and more, I see Western medicine treat way past the time of any meaningful relief.

I still remember being in the kitchen talking with my sister's fiancé asking him how he was doing. It was the look in his eyes. The fear and panic of facing the inevitable and not wanting to die. I completely understood him at that moment because he was so much like me. I was watching myself on death row in my final days when all appeals had been denied. Being in my early 20's, that just freaked me out. I stopped coming around.

He passed eight months later. My sister was his sole caregiver and was working fulltime. I asked her about it much later. She just talked about what happened and how she dealt with it. I told her why I stopped coming by. She never blamed me for not coming by. But I guess I do.

Learning to Listen

We all need connection and listening can be just the right messenger . -Kim

When the stress becomes overwhelming, caregivers and those being cared for need someone who can listen.

I don't know if we are born with listening skillsets. I imagine we were born with listening skillsets. Then life starts, and we forget that skillset. Or, our own experiences have us thinking we must do something more than listen.

A great tool exists called "active listening." In active listening, you can learn three or four skills that help you become a better listener and help you see when you are not listening. The skills help you know when you are making the conversation about you. The skills are so simple you can read a book on active listening and get the general gist of the process.

Even though the skills are simple, the process isn't because this is a confusing time. Caregiving is filled with your desire to make everything the best possible everything it could be. There are all sorts of things you may do that will be the opposite of active listening. Yet, every one of these things is based on the best intentions.

Here are some of the non-listening actions I've have seen and accidentally do. I've included why they might not help the person you are caring for cope with their situation, feel more empowered to make their decisions, or improve their resilience.

1.   When listening, you might feel an internal push to demonstrate understanding by sharing your own experiences and what was learned from your experiences. This may be the opposite of helping because your person may need to be heard. Getting sound advice about your life sounds more like a conversation about you.

2.   You may feel the need to help make decisions and start sharing your knowledge, opinion, or trivia. It always helps to check in first and validate that they want your advice. Otherwise, your well intention share may feel more like solutions for your life and not their solutions for their life.

3.   Sometimes we feel pressed to share our perspective on the situation. While you might feel

offering your insights will reduce their suffering, it may make them feel discounted and lessen the validity of their story.

4.   Your share may come from a desire to protect and safeguard a person. During listening, you assume the person will express some bad behavior that may cause them or another person harm. Suggesting, assuming, stating that the person sharing is going to act in a certain way can destroy trust. If you feel a need to warn against behaviors, check-in first, and verify that is even a thought in their head.

You never know what is going on in another person's head. Granted I was the caregiver, but people around you are participating. You will talk to them and share your observations or concerns. I found people have some seriously dark thoughts inside their head. The thoughts would take me by surprise. I would wonder, "Where the heck did that come from?" And my next thought would be "Pyscho."

Think before sharing your behavior warning and do a quick check to make sure it doesn't sound mean, nasty, super socially inappropriate. If it does and you can't see that before you share, then the person is justified in calling you a "Pyscho" and limiting future contact and communication.

As a caregiver, you may have so many beautiful intents and desires for the person you are taking care of. You may want the terminally ill patient to travel and experience the beauty of the world before life ends. For those who are sick or aging, there may be the desire for them to get better. There are the desires to have them stay here on earth. For our grandchildren, we may want them to grow up a healthy, independent person.

All your desires can pale against the need to be heard. Every caregiver and every person who finds themselves in a position to need a caregiver will need to be heard at some point. Caregiving means life has changed and sometimes in a problematic way.

Caregiving will present big decisions - decisions that must be made and usually quickly. There are uncomfortable emotions that are circling around your head. Life has lost some of its order and has become confusing. Critical pieces of your identity may become compromised.

Active listening works so well because it focuses on the person who is talking. Whether it is the caregiver or the one being cared for, they may have issues and emotions that they need to share. Active listening is formulated to build trust and demonstrate understanding. These two things can help develop a sense of empowerment, improve the ability to cope, and create greater resilience.

As a caregiver, I would highly recommend finding that one person in your group of friends who knows how to listen actively. Many people use counselors for this. If you can find a friend with this skillset, it will give you a much stronger coping mechanism. You will be able to get compassion closer to when you need compassion instead of when it is scheduled.

PART 2: Stress

I will breathe. I will not let my stress overwhelm me.

-    Kim

Why Stress isn't Treated Well in Western Medicine

Western pharmacopeia, the new gateway drug.

-    *Kim*

Western medicine has reached great heights treating the body like a car, a machine made with mechanical parts. All we need do is take apart the pieces and study the pieces. Like a car, when something isn't working, we can change the part. For Western medicine, replacing the part means using pharmaceuticals or surgery to change the body.

This has worked well for almost a full century. But diseases have become more cumbersome and lifestyles more hectic. Western medicine has served as a beacon of hope for some of the new infectious diseases of our time. Yet, Western medicine has shown little progress in addressing the chronic diseases of our time. Why is that?

The body isn't a car. When we tinker around with medications, we force different parts of the body to do something they don't want to do. The question becomes, "Is there a reason why these parts are acting this way? Do we know better than the body?"

That is a question I ask myself daily.

There are five unifying principles in biology. Unifying principles are fundamental truths that serve as the foundation for a system and the foundation for reasoning. Unifying principles in biology are believed to be true for all life. The flower, the bird, the human all adhere to the unifying principles of biology.

One of the five unifying principles of biology is homeostasis. Homeostasis is the ability of the body to maintain a constant internal environment in response to environmental changes such as external temperatures and humidity[9]. Homeostasis is how the body ensures survival.

---

[9] Bailey, R. (2017, March 6). What Is Homeostasis? Retrieved from https://www.thoughtco.com/homeostasis-defined-373304

Science states the nervous and endocrine systems control homeostasis in the body through feedback loops. The loops involve various hormones, chemicals, and organs[10]. Some examples of homeostatic processes are temperature controls, which keep us close to 98.6 Fahrenheit or 37 Celsius, or internal pH balance, water, and electrolyte balance, or blood pressure. Homeostasis suggests any disorder in the body is the body's attempt to survive.

A car does not have this type of intelligence. The different parts of the vehicle are needed for the whole unit to work, but parts can fail. The air conditioner can fail, and we can still drive the car. We can have an oil drip, and the car still runs. Each part of the vehicle is an independent, self-sufficient, self-contained unit. One part can be easily swapped for a new part.

Conversely, each aspect of the body is dependent on all other aspects of the body. A response in a distant area of the body will have a direct impact and can change the action of another part of the body. Changing

---

[10] Bailey, R. (2017, March 6). What Is Homeostasis? Retrieved from https://www.thoughtco.com/homeostasis-defined-373304

a reaction in the body with medications forces the body to stop doing what it believes it needs to do to survive and will cause internal stress.

What happens when a sandbag is removed from the dam? Water starts breaking through. Over time, the area around the missing sandbag starts to erode. More water comes through. Finally, there is a failure.

The pharmaceutical goal is to stop something in the body to suppress the symptom. The goal is not to heal the body. When have you gone to your doctor and heard them say,

"Oh yeah, that arthritis, I'm going to prescribe you this pill. I want you to take it for a month. At the end of the month, your symptoms should be gone, and you can stop taking the pill."

Never.

Here is another example, high blood pressure is a severe and widespread disease. When have you worked with your doctor to identify the cause of your high blood pressure and correct the cause so you won't need medications for the rest of your life?

Never.

Suppressing the symptom isn't always a bad option. Pain is a symptom experienced by so many of us.

We are aware of how uncomfortable pain is and how much relief we can get from a Tylenol or aspirin. At times, this type of symptom elimination is a huge benefit.

Sometimes pain management is not a huge benefit, especially in chronic pain management. In my practice, I have seen clients who come in with chronic long-term back pain. They have been using Western pharmacy for years to manage the pain. For some of these clients, they had graduated to managing their pain with OxyContin.

OxyContin is an opioid used for the management of pain severe enough to require daily treatment. It is one of the most potent painkillers we have and has a high rate of addiction.

The problem with OxyContin is that it turns off the pain sensors. Remember, homeostasis is the need to protect the body to survive? Pain is one way the body helps protect an area of the body that has been damaged. With the suppression of the pain symptom, you can continue to use your body but will cause continuous damage.

At some point and time, the OxyContin is going to stop working, and there will be breakthrough pain.

How much damage has happened for the pain to break through our most potent pain killer?

When I first started seeing patients who had been using opioids for years and were experiencing breakthrough pain, I would try and treat them. Treating them never worked out.

My objective tools, such as a force gauge (tests the pounds exerted on the area before feeling pain) or goniometer (measures the joint range of motion), indicated the client was making statistically significant improvements.

Here is the problem. Pain scales are commonly a scale of 1-10, with 10 being that the pain is so bad, you can't get out of bed. Each person has a different tolerance. Most patients prescribed OxyContin are at a 10. Think about how bad the pain is after years of opioid use, and the patient has breakthrough pain. Sometimes doctors want to explain away the increasing levels of pain as building up a tolerance to the drug. And tolerance can explain a reduction in sensitivity to opioids. Yet, Western medicine hasn't been able to prove tolerance is the sole issue or even most of the problem for break-thru pain. Drugs reduce our body's ability to respond and manage pain.

In my practice, people who have long term Opioid use for pain usually can no longer reduce pain to a manageable level through acupuncture. A standard pain scale rates pain on a scale of 1-10, with 10 being unable to get out of bed. If their suffering was a 10 before OxyContin and after years of using opioids, the pain is back, my clinical experience suggests increased damage to the area.

It appears that breakthrough pain is no longer on the standard pain scale. So, let's just say your pain is a 15. Well, even if I could reduce it by 5 points to a 10, it would still be unbearable and be unacceptable.

I use the example of pain because we all have experienced pain and can easily relate to it. If homeostasis is accurate and the Western science of Biology thinks homeostasis is a unifying principle, then suppressing the symptom of pain would force the body to adjust unnaturally.

The second question I think, "Are the side effects of the medications due to the medications or due to the body being forced to act unnaturally?"

If I'm to believe in science, my gut reaction is that the side effects are due to the medications forcing the body to behave in unnatural ways. Because the drugs are not fixing the problem or the symptom, the expression needs to find another way out. When I think about finding another way out, I think about the natural disaster of flooding. In a flood, that is what water does...it finds another way out. Thus, the side effects.

Here is another example of stress on the body: acid indigestion. Omeprazole, also known as Prilosec, is a standard method of reducing heartburn pain. The problem with Prilosec or Omeprazole is the medication does not help to resolve the original issue of acid indigestion.

Every patient of mine who has taken a Protein Pump Inhibitor like Omeprazole long-term report their symptoms gradually increase over time. Like water backing up behind the dam, the pressure continues to mount. They report higher sensitivity to more and more foods.

Let's look at the dam analogy further. Rain continues to fall, threatening to crest the dam. We start to add sandbags to the dam just as my patients report taking more Omeprazole. Finally, the pressure of the water begins to overwhelm the dam. The dam starts to show cracks, and water starts finding its way through the dam just as my patients report breakthrough acid reflux with almost anything they eat. For many patients, coffee and bread are significant contributors to acid reflux.

When the acid reflux has reached the point where it is breaking through the medications, it is difficult and requires significant patient participation to fix. The hectic pace of life can be overwhelming, and the extensive patient participation needed to correct acid reflux is frustrating. The need for the involvement is probably more frustrating because Western medicine was selling the belief they had a pill that would fix everything. Acid reflux can be the first time a patient is faced with the fact there isn't a pill to fix anything. For myself, it wasn't until I ended up in the Emergency Room with level 10 pain that I changed my lifestyle. The only thing that kept me honest was any deviation from what I needed to do with food caused an immediate level 10 pain, which would take days to eliminate. You can watch my whole experience on my YouTube channel @bestacupuncturellc. Look for the "30 Day Challenge" series.

The second concern with Western pharmacopeia is the side effects. Every medication has a side effect that will be treated with another drug that has a different side effect that can be treated with another medicine.

Omeprazole is a key cause of low magnesium levels[11] and impaired bone remodeling[12]. Fosamax is the standard medication to improve bone density and bone remodeling. Yet, Fosamax has been shown to have reduced efficacy with Omeprazole and has also been proven to increase the potential risk for esophageal cancer, risk of thigh bone (femur) fractures, debilitating bone and muscle pain and risk of atrial fibrillation according to the FDA[13].

---

[11] Thongon, N., Penguy, J., Kulwong, S., Khongmueang, K., & Thongma, M. (2016). *Omeprazole suppressed plasma magnesium level and duodenal magnesium absorption in male Sprague-Dawley rats. Omeprazole suppressed plasma magnesium level and duodenal magnesium absorption in male Sprague-Dawley rats.* European Journal of Physiology. Retrieved from https://www.ncbi.nlm.nih.gov/pubmed/27866273

[12] Al Subaie, A., Emami, E., Tamimi, I., Laurenti, I., Eimar, H., Abdallah, M. N., & Tamimi, F. (2016). *Systemic administration of Omeprazole interferes with bone healing and implant osseointegration: an in vivo study on rat tibiae. Systemic administration of Omeprazole interferes with bone healing and implant osseointegration: an in vivo study on rat tibiae.* Journal of Clinical Periodontology. Retrieved from https://www.ncbi.nlm.nih.gov/pubmed/26725944

[13] Fosamax: Uses, Dosage & How to Take Alendronate

So, did the medications cause the side effects, or did suppressing the symptom cause the side effect? Magnesium is critical for bone remodeling. Does reducing the stomach acid cause the reduction in magnesium uptake or increase elimination of magnesium, or does the medicine? I don't know. One thought could be that magnesium can only attach to a protein in the body at a specific pH level. The stomach is supposed to have a pH of 2.0 – or very acidic.

When we use a protein pump inhibitor, we inhibit gastric acid production or stop the symptom, but at what cost. Does the symptom find another way of expressing itself like water in a flood? In this case, the medications reduce gastric acid raising the pH of the stomach. Magnesium uptake is pH-dependent. So, for this situation, the drug is proven to cause the side effect of reduced bone remodeling. Yet, the point is, you still have horrible acid reflux, and now you bone remodeling issues. Makes Western pharmacy look like a gateway drug.

Sodium. (n.d.). Retrieved from
https://www.drugwatch.com/fosamax/

The concept of homeostasis is my first concern with trying to manage stress with Western medicine. If homeostasis is correct, suppressing symptoms will not fix the problem. It will cause more severe issues down the line.

But homeostasis isn't the only concern I have with using Western medicine for stress management. Stress has so many symptoms. When we look at the list of symptoms associated with the beginning stages of stress, they paint an interesting picture. Let's look at some of these symptoms:

Some of the most common symptoms experienced early on with stress will be:

· Fatigue and low energy,

· Headaches,

· Upset stomach including heartburn, acid reflux, nausea,

· Constipation or diarrhea,

· Pain such as muscle pain,

· Chest pain, rapid heartbeat,

· Insomnia

· Frequent colds and infections,

· Loss of sexual drive,

· Depression,

· Anxiety,

· Anger,

· Confusion,

· Difficulty understanding problems or situations,

· Inability to focus

These symptoms fall under a category considered as medically unexplained physical symptoms (MUPS). They are symptoms where, after adequate evaluation, a cause for the symptom may not be medically determined[14].

It is not unusual for a patient with MUPS to see their physician multiple times a year. A Dutch research survey looked at how many patients with four or more physician visits a year were visiting for MUPS. The study found that 2.5% of the patient load was MUPS patients[15].

---

[14] Henningsen, P., Zipfel, S., & Herzog, W. (2007). Management of functional somatic syndromes. *The Lancet, 369*(9565), 946–955. doi: 10.1016/s0140-6736(07)60159-7

[15] Hartman, T. O., Hassink-Franke, L., Dowrick, C., Fortes, S., Lam, C., Horst, H. V. D., ... Weel-Baumgarten, E. V. (2008). Medically unexplained symptoms in family medicine: defining a research agenda. Proceedings from

The difficulty with MUPS is traditional treatment. Traditional treatment for MUPS is doing nothing. Thus, Western medicine is a poor first choice for dealing with stress since most of the initial symptoms are MUPS. The typical physician response is to try and reassure the patient. The other problem is that people with multiple unexplained physical symptoms can look sick. If you look and feel sick, how come you can't get treatment.

MUPS are part of most diseases. You can see every one of these symptoms in cancer or IBS or congestive heart failure. They are common to all and specific to none. This suggests that stress may be the root of all disease. Just how common MUPS are can be seen in the studies done on MUPS. In England, a study indicated that about 33% of new neurological patients had symptoms consistent with MUPS[16].

WONCA 2007. *Family Practice, 25*(4), 266–271. doi: 10.1093/fampra/cmn041

[16] Kirsch, I., Deacon, B. J., Huedo-Medina, T. B., Scoboria, A., Moore, T. J., & Johnson, B. T. (2008). Initial Severity and Antidepressant Benefits: A Meta-Analysis of Data Submitted to the Food and Drug Administration. *PLoS Medicine, 5*(2). doi: 10.1371/journal.pmed.0050045

For long-term caregivers, the chronic nature of stress starts out with little or no pathology. After years of caregiving, the symptoms are severe and unique enough to identify a disease. Some of the common ones experienced by long-term caregivers are:

· acid reflux, heartburn turning into ulcers,

· headaches turning into migraines,

· high blood pressure,

· hypo-glycemia turning into diabetes,

· insomnia,

· anxiety turning into panic attacks,

If MUPS may be the root of all disease, wouldn't it make sense to try and figure out how to heal the signs of stress when they first start? If Western medicine wants us to wait until the symptoms become a disease, won't that make it much more difficult to cure?

The last aspect of Western medicine that I want to touch on is the placebo effect. In Western medicine, the placebo effect is a treatment with no predetermined therapeutic value producing a beneficial or healing effect in the body. Irving Kirsch has been a prolific placebo effect researcher. In 2008, he released a study that indicated the placebo effect was the same as medication[9]. Some researchers suggest the placebo effect could be worth as much as 30-50% of the total impact of the treatment.

In most research today, a placebo-controlled group is not used. Instead, the currently acceptable treatment is the comparison or control group. Yet, if the placebo effect can be such an active player in health, wouldn't you want to know how that stacks up to current treatment? Wouldn't you want to see why the mind and body can heal the person without medical intervention? Wouldn't the placebo effect be one of the most significant potential breakthroughs in modern medicine? Wouldn't you want your doctor to have more than 19 minutes of one class dedicated to the placebo effect? For me, the placebo effect is such an exciting topic and really brings into question our role in our own healing. How much do we own our well-being because the placebo effect seems to suggest we own a lot?

So, we have homeostasis. We have MUPS. We have the placebo effect. Homeostasis suggests unfavorable changes in the body are a survival adaption. MUPS indicates that stress may be the root of all disease. And the placebo effect suggests we play an active role in our healing. Whether you want to use Western medicine or not to help with your stress, science supports doing more than just Western medicine.

The Thing About Stress

"I just remember how noisy it got and suddenly it was just quiet..."

-Kim on remembering the end

The thing about stress is stress is different for everyone. How we experience stress, how we respond to stress, how stress initially shows up in the body, why stress shows up where it shows up is about the individuality of the human body.

The thing not unique about stress is the impact on the body. Stress is cumulative. The longer stress goes on, the more symptoms appear, the more force stress ~~applies to the body, and the~~ more pronounced impact

[17] Karlstrom, K. E., Lee, J. P., Kelley, S. A., Crow, R. S., Crossey, L. J., Young, R. A., ... Shuster, D. L. (2014). Formation of the Grand Canyon 5 to 6 million years ago through integration of older palaeocanyons. *Nature Geoscience, 7*(3), 239–244. doi: 10.1038/ngeo2065

each successive stressor has on the body. Stress reminds me of the persistent patience of water.

How long did it take the Colorado River to create the Grand Canyon? Maybe six million years[17]. I don't really know that six million years is a true number. The point is the number is a really big number. Throughout the whole time, water just kept moving. It just kept moving as soft as rain or as forceful as spring flooding. It just kept on being water. At no time did water change course or even ponder its impact on the canyon. With each successive year, the canyon got deeper and deeper lulling more water to flow down the same path creating fissures within the rock. Fatiguing the rock until it finally broke or wore away.

Stress is like water. Stress has patience and persistence. It cares little for its impact on the body and like dredging a canyon, each successive stressor can dredge a deeper and deeper canyon in our physical well-being, fatiguing us, breaking us down.

I like the definition of fatigue used in Materials Science when thinking about stress in the human body.

"fatigue is the weakening of a material caused by repeatedly applied loads. It is the progressive and localized structural damage that occurs when a material

*is subjected to cyclic loading. The nominal maximum **stress** values that cause such damage may be much less than the strength of the material "*

Wow. I don't know if every caregiver will experience this. I just know I have yet to meet a caregiver not experiencing the damage caused by stress.

The person doesn't even have to be holding down the "caregiver" role. They may be participating in other ways. They may be trying to support the primary caregiver. Even supportive roles, which seem like they would be so much more minor, can have a serious impact on the person because stress just doesn't care.

After my role as caregiver had ceased, the implications of caregiver stress became real. I was trying to meditate. I couldn't quiet my mind. I couldn't even come close to quieting my mind. I became aware of a base layer of noise that was constantly humming inside of me. A nervous anxiety. Any minor inconvenience became a mountain. I would start to ruminate over the problem blowing the problem up like a balloon until it finally popped in my head. I had difficulty completing tasks and found tasks to be exhausting or overwhelming.

I had weird physical symptoms.

- My tongue would hurt. The pain would become a chronic burning pain making it difficult to eat.

- I never get headaches. I was getting headaches. The headaches were dull and last days.

- My vision would blur making it hard to read a book. I couldn't keep my attention while reading making it difficult to read a paragraph.

- I couldn't sleep. If I went to sleep, I would wake up multiple times and not be able to get back to sleep.

- I was getting pain all over my body.

My emotions were out of control. I was getting angry over everything. I was so sad. The grief was so overwhelming. I would sit and cry for hours. I was depressed and didn't want people around me. I started avoiding people. I was experiencing panic attacks.

Moreover, I became acutely aware that even very small stressors would start to trigger a cacophony of stress responses in me. Having a disagreement became so much more than a disagreement. I started questioning my daily actions and reactions.

"The nominal maximum stress values that cause such damage may be much less than the strength of the material ..."

I thought I had been so much stronger than the situations I was in. In my life, I had survived and thrived in difficult environments. Caregiving was different. There were so many situations happening at one time. And, I was so worn down. It took very little now to become overwhelmed.

I had a clinical understanding of PTSD. I was getting a real-life experience on what PTSD really meant. Empathy takes on a whole new meaning when you have your own real-life experience.

Stress In the body

90% of what is stressing you today will be irrelevant in a year.

Long-term chronic stress in the body is always detrimental. Everyone experiences stress differently. People will have a similar end-stage experience. How you got there can take many different paths.

When I think about how Chinese Medicine looks at the individual, I think about math and how math gives meaning to our environment through formulas that help define our world.

The formula that sticks in my head when thinking about the many paths an individual can take to get to the same place is a permutation. In permutations, every detail matter. Details change the answer. A Chimpanzee has a genome that is estimated to be only 1.2% different from humans[18]. The difference between individual humans averages 0.1%[19].

Permutations look at all the possible ways of doing something and deliver an answer. For life to have enough similar characteristics that it can be defined as a species that can interbreed, it has less than a 0.1% variance in DNA.

---

[18] How Do We Know Humans Are Primates? (2018, June 27). Retrieved from http://humanorigins.si.edu/education/how-do-we-know/how-do-we-know-humans-are-primates

[19] One Species, Living Worldwide. (2019, January 15). Retrieved from http://humanorigins.si.edu/evidence/genetics/one-species-living-worldwide

Wow, and look at what that 0.1% delivers. We have different skin colors, different heights, different IQ's, different voice, eye color, weight, and on and on and on. In all the world of 6 billion people, each of us is unique from every other person. And all that came from only a 0.1% variance in DNA.

In Chinese medicine, differences matter. That is why one disease can have many different paths and be treated in many ways. How you got to your disease is unique from every other individual on the planet. Yet, the result may look the same. Isn't that amazing?

O.k., so everyone is different with a similar result. So what? When we look at stress, there are some common physical symptoms that many of us experience. The initial symptoms associated with stress are common to almost every disease out there. Which is unusual in that it suggests stress could be a leading factor to illness. As the experience of stress is prolonged are symptoms increase and can gradually progress to disease.

Going back to permutations and Chinese medicine, every detail matters. You won't get all the symptoms associated with stress, but you will get some of them. And some of the symptoms will be more severe than others. Based on your unique permutation, you can focus on some specific areas and use particular strategies to help you manage your stress.

Some of the most common symptoms experienced early on with stress will be:

· Fatigue and low energy,

· Headaches,

· Upset stomach including heartburn, acid reflux, nausea, gas, bloating,

· Constipation or diarrhea,

· Pain such as muscle pain,

· Chest pain, rapid heartbeat,

· Insomnia

· Frequent colds and infections,

· Loss of sexual drive,

· Depression,

· Anxiety,

· Anger,

· Confusion,

· Difficulty understanding problems or situations,

· Inability to focus

It is not unusual to find caregivers in their role for five or more years. With prolonged stress, health deteriorates, and the symptoms become more severe. Due to the increasing age of caregivers, it is more likely their health will deteriorate quicker. Some of the more severe symptoms can include:

· Weight gain or obesity,

· Ulcers,

· Spastic colon,

· Irritable bowel syndrome,

· Fiber myalgia,

· Chronic fatigue,

· Asthma,

· Diabetes,

· Migraines,

· High blood pressure,

· High cholesterol,

· Heart disease,

· Panic Attacks and Agoraphobia,

· Gallstones,

· Pancreatitis,

Stress…

It's likely you will get to see some of these in yourself and may get to see some of them in people you are caring for.

At all stages, the fatigue is real. The emotions are real. There can always be self-doubt and blame. One of the most common avoidance tactics I've seen in practice and in my personal life is the drive to keep busy. Busy, busy, busy... If you are busy, you don't have time to feel all the emotions swirling inside of you. In Chinese Medicine, the organ channel which we most commonly use to drive and propel ourselves forward even when we are exhausted is the liver channel.

I had one patient; we had gotten most of her symptoms under control. My belief was that grief over the loss of one of her family members was causing her symptoms. I thought the root of her disease was in her lung channel. If we got rid of everything blocking the lung channel, everything would be fine. Clearing everything that was blocking the expression of the lung channel was working.

Her symptoms indicated the energy of the liver was overwhelming, and stopping the energy of the lung channel. I put her on a formula geared to her specific symptoms.

When she came in the following week, she was so sad and dejected. She had downcast eyes and didn't feel like doing anything. I was so confused. These were not liver symptoms. Why did she suddenly exhibit all these lung symptoms?

It took me a little bit of time and looking at the Five Element theory on Qi movement to finally realize what had happened. The formula had worked as expected. In Chinese Medicine, the liver is viewed as "The General" and oversees activity and action. Many people facing trying emotional issues, life-threatening diseases suddenly go into a flurry of activity to distract themselves. My patient was doing precisely that. She was in a flurry of activity to avoid the enormous grief she was experiencing. The formula put her liver back in balance and allowed her lung energy to express itself finally.

Without her crutch, all her emotions of grief, confusion, dismay, hurt came rushing forward. One of the bummers with grief is it is something you must go through. Having healthy lungs and a working large intestine will make the process easier. But you still must process grief to get through it.

Cancer patients are another one where you will see them pushing through things and ignoring their body to avoid the emotions.

And in people who are experiencing a lot of stress as a caregiver, you will find that they use the liver to push them past their actual energy level to avoid the emotions and strain of caregiving and just to get things done.

The one positive thing about the energy of the liver is it can help distract and protect you. In Chinese medicine, the liver, as "The General," also has a crucial responsibility of protecting and defending you. In Western medicine, the liver's responsibility for detoxing is the responsibility of protecting and safeguarding your body. With the emotions, distraction through activity becomes the liver's expression.

On the other side, one of the key emotions of the liver is kindness, and it is an act of kindness to distract you from the many woes of life, especially when you don't have the strength to face them.

Yet, back to my patient. Grief is a process that you must walk through all by yourself. But, just like Chinese Medicine can put your liver back in balance, Chinese Medicine can support the lungs to help them stay in balance during the grieving process ensuring your grief doesn't become pathogenic.

PART 3: Why Chinese Medicine

The field is the sole governing agency of the particle.

-   Albert Einstein

The question is, "Why use Chinese Medicine"?[20][21][22] A significant reason to use Chinese Medicine is the medicine offers to heal you. Healing is a big difference.

How does Chinese Medicine heal you? Chinese Medicine accepts the whole body as an active

[20] Aung, S. K., Fay, H., & Hobbs, R. F. (2013). Traditional Chinese Medicine as a Basis for Treating Psychiatric Disorders: A Review of Theory with Illustrative Cases. *Medical Acupuncture, 25*(6), 398–406. doi: 10.1089/acu.2013.1007

[21] Tan, C., Chen, W., Wu, Y., & Chen, S. (2013). Chinese medicine for mental disorder and its applications in psychosomatic diseases. *Chinese Medicine for Mental Disorder and Its Applications in Psychosomatic Diseases, 19*(1), 59–69.

[22] Yuan, T. F. (2009). Traditional Chinese Medicine in treatments to depression. *Neuro Endrocrinology Letters, 30*(1).

participant in health. If every part of the body is doing their job, everything will be o.k. It's when one part of the body changes and its task start going sideways.

Weakening the function of the liver is very easy to do today. It is estimated that 66% of the U.S. adult population [23] uses prescription drugs. Prescription drugs and ibuprofen are two opportunities to weaken the liver. The liver is responsible for detoxing the medications from our system. Add drinking alcohol, and we've probably covered a good percentage of the U.S. adult population.

It is easier to impair liver function because we are unaware that we are creating a problem. We are having so much fun eating tasty foods, having the excitement of the emotional ups and downs of life, and a whole lot of other things. Stopping and reversing the process of impairment is much more complicated than getting to liver impairment.

When Western medicine identifies a disease, there is some suggestions organ function may be

---

[23] Georgetown University. (n.d.). Prescription Drugs. Retrieved from https://hpi.georgetown.edu/agingsociety/pubhtml/rxdrugs/rxdrugs.html

dropped to 30%. So, we have partied through 70% of our organ function before Western medicine raises the warning flag. Add to that, organ function deteriorates as we age, and just living would impact our overall health.

Every organ in the body depends on the liver in some way. The liver stores sugar. If storing sugars is impaired, the bloodstream will have more sugars circulating, which can lead to diabetes. Diabetes tends to damage the small blood vessels of the body. When the small blood vessels in the kidneys are injured, the kidneys start retaining more water and salt. Salt and water retention can lead to weight gain, high blood pressure, and the process will go on and on. Maybe the next organ impacted could be the heart.

It is easy to impair organ function today, and, it appears, it was easy to reduce organ function in ancient China. Ancient China just took a different path to understanding health.

Here is a little folklore that helps to point out the difference between our Western medicine and medicine in ancient China. In Ancient China, they say the doctor would get paid if the patient remained healthy. The patient had to do what the doctor told them to do. If the patient did as told and got sick, the doctor would have to pay the patient. Today, it seems this method would leave a lot of poor doctors and wealthy patients. Just think, some of us wouldn't have to work. We would get so much money from our doctors. Yet, that is just an example of how Chinese Medicine took a different path to health.

Another way Ancient China differs from Western Medicine is the goal in Chinese Medicine is to improve health instead of trying to force the body to pretend everything is o.k.

Western prescription medicines basically work by forcing the body to change some function in the body. Statins work by inhibiting the function of HMG-CoA reductase[24], a key enzyme responsible for the manufacture of cholesterol. Omeprazole works as a selective and irreversible proton pump inhibitor[25]. The

---

[24] Stancu, C., & Sima, A. (2001). Statins: mechanism of action and effects. *Journal of Cellular and Molecular Medicine, 5*(4), 378–387. doi: 10.1111/j.1582-4934.2001.tb00172.x

[25] B, W., P, L., & Larsson, H. (1985). The mechanism of action of omeprazole—a survey of its inhibitory actionsin vitro. *Scandinavian Journal of Gastroenterology, 20*(sup108), 37–51. doi: 10.3109/00365528509095818

proton pump is responsible for creating acids in the stomach. Other medications work by encouraging the body to produce more of a response. Oxycodone and OxyContin attach to the opioid receptor in the brain and fire off the receptor. Opioid receptors are responsible for blocking pain and producing a calming effect when fired.

The point is much Western medicine is focused on making the body behave in a manner different than how the body wants to act.

Western Medicine offers a beguiling suggestion of a quick fix. The medications can have an immediate effect until they don't. Omeprazole works until it doesn't. And when it stops working, the stomach acid reflux has graduated from bad to unbearable. The deceptive quick fix Omeprazole offered lures us into a false sense of security. Everything seems alright until it isn't.

On the other hand, Chinese Medicine is focused on improving the natural function of the body. By supporting and strengthening the innate capacity, the body organically corrects the imbalance. In Chinese Medicine, the issue can take time, and you must participate.

When it comes to the stomach, the stomach takes a solid effort and a lot of participation. You might need to reduce food intake, eliminate foods, take herbs, and use acupuncture. To fix a health issue through Chinese Medicine is always more involved than taking a pill.

Although, in the end, Chinese Medicine can leave you feeling great and may leave you living without medications. In Western Medicine, you still feel stressed and overwhelmed.

I remember watching the old Kungfu movies. You might remember them. Where the actor's mouth moves much faster than the words and remains moving far after the words stopped coming through your speakers. In the movies, the hero is about finding longevity and power. Longevity is a life well-lived. Power is letting go of attachments. The hero found their center in patience and through managing their mind and their body. They found it by sitting down and locating all the disturbed and distributed parts of themselves and bringing them back together. They found it through the integration of the body, mind, emotions, and spirit.

All that sounds spiritual and way beyond the time and patience we have in our already hectic lives.

Yet, Chinese Medicine is about training the body and mind to use each part evenly. With every treatment, your body is introduced to a new possibility of reacting. Chinese Medicine has many different tools and methods to train your body and mind almost without your conscious recognition.

It's not like going to counseling, where you spend years trying to process all the stress and emotions you experienced. It's not like going to a physician and getting medications that can numb the feelings. Chinese Medicine is about helping the body remember what it was like to be healthy and how to let go of disease.

Can Chinese Medicine really help you let go of disease?

Part of Chinese medicine is the concept everything that happens in this life is mapped somewhere on the body. You might be aware of the physical symptom, but in Chinese Medicine, the physical manifestation is only part of the disease.

You go to school to learn a skill like Information Technology, Business Administration, Engineering. To learn that skill takes a lot of time. You spend 12 years preparing the basics in elementary, middle, and high school. Then you test to see if you have done enough to get accepted at another training institute that will let you train even more for the career you want. You spend another 2 to 8 years studying for a profession.

You have spent time learning about a profession and very little time learning about ourselves. Your mind, emotions, and body have been allowed free reign. They have expressed themselves with no regard for the rest of the body.

School is not necessarily mental training. School teaches you how to memorize things, take tests, apply logic. What it doesn't do is help you think through life situations and daily events with grace. Instead, the pressure to succeed has caused many imbalances within the mind and body.

Chinese medicine offers the training, tools, and technics to start pulling it all together and healing yourself. The focus isn't on one aspect of the person. The focus isn't on one symptom. The medicine is about making you stronger by identifying areas of weakness or blocks and treating them to strengthen weakness and open blocks.

The Key Concept is Integration

The state of your life can reflect the state of your mind.

-Kim

Chinese Medicine has always focused on finding the best balance within yourself.

Daoist and Buddhist monks appeared to go about their daily activities with so much peace and inner grace. I wondered how they did it. How did they walk around with so much harmony and inner peace? How were they able to view the disruption that happens in the world and see a neutral side of the chaos? Maybe it was an act. But, if the walk wasn't an act, how were they able to do it?

Finding an answer to the question of internal harmony and peace wasn't clear, but I found guidance in Classical Chinese Medicine.

The concept of integration is a foundation in Chinese Medicine. Everything is related to everything in the body. The environment, your mental attitude, your emotions, your genetic inheritance, and your physical body all interact and respond to each other. Chinese Medicine asks to respect each aspect and work with it to flourish. You lack wisdom when you ignore the interrelatedness of your body, your lives, and your universe.

In Western Medicine, a little is known about integration in the body with words like homeostasis. Homeostasis defines the body's attempt to stay in balance and survive. It does this through complicated signaling mechanisms. One of the more well-known signaling mechanisms is the signal your body gives when you try to diet and eat less food. Your body protects you by reducing your metabolic functions. So much for the diet. As your metabolic function gets out of balance, conditions like diabetes, high blood pressure, fatigue, nausea, etc. start showing up.

In Chinese Medicine, it is more than just the physical body. It is the physical body, the thought processes, the emotions, the genetic inheritance, lifestyle, and environment, which all make up the health and well-being of an individual.

Each of these parts is integrated. If one part is impacted, all parts will slowly weaken and become predisposed to illness.

The stress in caregiving impacts every aspect of the body. All the emotions involved in caregiving and the intensity of the feelings can have you on high alert. Because caregiving can be 24x7, you don't get many options to get away and have personal time. And trying to stay healthy becomes a more significant challenge.

The scientific studies on stress in the body start to play out in your life. Long-term stress isolates the caregiver from other people. Although one way to cope and deal with stress is through your friendships and talking, in caregiving, you have less and less time for other people. With less time for others, you might find fewer people in your life. A critical method for managing stress can be lost with the loss of people in your life.

You don't just lose time for other people; you lose time for yourself and your own self-care. Sure, as people age, they tend to need more care. Yet, having to manage your life and another's life, you may find you are just too tired to do anything - even if that means sleep.

You become isolated and disconnected from yourself. It could be your craving for friendships, your need for that 1 hour of personal time. It could be anything. You just don't get it. Instead, you feel you must push yourself more and more to get things done.

The integration focus of Classical Chinese medicine helps you reconnect the different parts of your

body one step at a time. Any of the tools or theories
help with this. When you are focusing on stress and
trying to find self-care, a simple understanding of Five
Element Theory and nature can let you use Chinese
medical options to give relief to your stress.

Focus Is on The Whole Body

You are more than your body.

-Kim

Caregiving isn't just a title or role which you put
on and then take off at the end of the day. Caregiving
becomes a lifestyle that impacts every part of the body.
An example could be the chronic stress slowly elevating
the blood pressure. Secondary symptoms such as
diarrhea, poor appetite, heartburn, insomnia, and
nervous energy can also appear.

Western pharmacopia masks the symptoms, and
you continue to get sicker. Sometimes, only masking a
symptom is a good thing. When the metal pins in my
mom's knee finally broke at age 81, and she started
having knee pain and swelling, masking the pain with
cortisone injections and drawing out the excess fluids

was a very valid option. She was pass fixing it. Yet, you are not usually at that point when you are caregivers.

Instead, you are at a point where you could still have a long productive life. Part of that is going to depend on how you come through your time as a caregiver. If you focus solely on using Western medicine to get through the strain of caregiving, there are good chances that at the end of your time as a caregiver, you may be too sick to have any desire to improve your life.

For many of us, the end of caregiving comes so abruptly that all our drive forward suddenly has no opposing force. The abrupt end cascades into a valley of emotional turmoil. What you learn and how you manage the stress of caregiving will be useful for the rest of our life.

The Focus on Nature

Of all the paths you take in life, make sure a few of them are dirt.

-John Muir

What I really like about Chinese Medicine is the connection with nature. I grew up in a little farming community where nature was a part of my daily life. I remember playing in the grove or climbing trees or lying in the grass watching the big, fluffy cumulus clouds float by like a thousand ships across a crystal blue sea. I can remember the heat of summer engulfed in sounds of crickets and the humid, sweaty nights drenched in the hum of mosquitos. I grew up at a time where GMO crops were starting to coming in, and farmers were still saving their seeds for next season's planting. We walked our fields to eliminate weeds.

There was always a peacefulness in nature and a quietness that brought about a level of solitude and comfort. I can remember the end of a summer day when the sun was starting to fade. The heat would weigh down the land. I would go for long walks down narrow dirt roads that ended nowhere in the middle of the fields to sit and watch the sunset.

I always had a connection to nature. Later, I moved into the big cities. When my world became too stressful, I would jump in my car and drive out into nature to find a place to sit, quiet my mind, and eliminate my stress. I would grab my backpack and head into the canyons or forests for a few days to find peace.

When Chinese Medicine came along, the medicine validated what I had felt for most of my life…a unity between us and nature.

What was taught in Chinese medical school was the verbiage of heaven above, earth below, and humans in between. It was simple and resonated with our interpretation of being human. The heavens above give us energy. The earth below provides a foundation. You stand in between the two. We see ourselves as independent and justified in using things to our own advancement. In fact, we have a sort of "Manifest Destiny" belief the world is here to support us, and it is our right to use the world as we see fit. The deeper I investigated Chinese Medicine, the more complicated the concept became, and the more misguided a human-centric view of the world became.

The obvious interpretation of heaven/human/earth was the current physical existence between heaven and earth. Yet, there was more to it than just that. The trilogy was a model that described one thing…life. Which meant that although we see ourselves today as separate from heaven and earth, in truth, we are a unity of heaven, earth, and human. The trilogy becomes one thing, and our life only exists because heaven and earth are here.

A simple way of looking at it is to look at oxygen. Oxygen in the heavens sustains your life. Food or water from the earth sustains your lives. Oxygen from the heavens, food and water from the earth is viewed as separate. Your skin is an imaginary boundary separating you from the world. Skin allows you to think you are independent of your surroundings.

Chinese Medicine views this in a slightly different light. The very oxygen that permeates your lungs is the same oxygen, which saturates your environment. The winds, the plants, the oceans move oxygen throughout the world just as blood vessels, lungs, heart move oxygen throughout the body.

The blood vessels distribute oxygen to the different parts of the body, enabling various cells to uptake needed oxygen. Just as the winds, the plants, the oceans distribute oxygen throughout the world with different lifeforms taking oxygen as required.

The concept of "as above so below" became more understandable. What was happening above was happening below. So, just looking at the example of oxygen, just as the planet moves oxygen to ensure that every cell that needs oxygen can get oxygen, the body moves oxygen, providing the cells that need the oxygen get it.

The boundaries we create seem to have allowed us to compartmentalize our world and maybe make it more understandable. Yet, the boundaries also granted the ability to create separation. Separation enabled justification to use the world to satiate immediate desires with little regard for the long-term implications.

The separation supported a belief that actions were not interdependent. Yet, we are only here because we have the heavens above and the earth below. If those things are here and can support life, we will continue to survive. This interdependence also touches on the health of life…all of life…the trilogy of life. Only if all parts are healthy can we be healthy.

From this conversation, one of the concepts of nature in Chinese Medicine is based on interdependence and unity.

There is another way in which nature is used in Chinese Medicine. Concepts are explained through nature. One of the fundamental principles in Chinese Medicine is the 12 organ channels/meridians. Many have an understanding of the 12 channels in Chinese

Medicine. Each of the 12 channels/meridians is associated with a body organ. Six of the organs/channels are yin, and six of the organs/channels are yang. These channels transverse the body from the toes to the head. What most people don't know about these channels or meridians is that Chinese Medicine describes the channels as waterways.

In ancient China, the waterways were critical. Some of their functions included: distributing nutrients, normalizing temperatures, removing debris, and repairing the earth. The birthplace of China is in the valley of the Yellow River, one of the two great rivers in China. The Yellow River is the most fertile land in China and is prone to flooding. In the 1931 flooding, It is stated millions may have died. To this day, the Yellow River is prone to flooding.

One of the Five Ancient Emperors (before 2070 B.C.) is reported to have incorporated irrigation to help better manage the Yellow River and reduce the flooding. These changes ensured better health and longer life for the population.

In Chinese Medicine, the 12 channels are part of the waterways of our body. Their energy starts at the tips of the fingers and toes. Chinese Medicine has 360 points to learn. Some of the points are categorized into groups of functionality. The transport points are one category. The name implies an essential function of waterways to transport something.

There are 5 transport points on each channel. Depending on the channel, the points will either start at the fingers or start at the toes. Half of the channels begin at the toes; half of the channels start at the fingers. Here is an example. The liver channel begins at the toes and ends at the ribs. The small intestine channel begins at the fingertips and ends at the ear.

The 5 transport points have a name describing the strength of the Qi at the spot. The five names are: well, spring, stream, river, sea. A well is deep and quiet, waiting to be brought to the surface. The water bubbles forth in a spring that trickles towards a stream. The streams join to make a river. Rivers gather strength and flow to large bodies of water, such as seas.

Just as ancient China used irrigation to manage the Yellow River, so acupuncturists use the concepts of irrigation to use these five points better and improve the health of the individual.

The use of nature in Chinese Medicine helped define the Five Element theory in Chinese Medicine.

Five Elements is about energy and movement. It uses nature to help identify the energetics involved and the universal order. The five elements are Fire, Earth, Metal, Water, Wood.

The five elements are represented in the body by an "official." The official is designated to one of five yin organs in the body.

Five Element defines many things. There are three things which Five Element theory describes and pertain to this discussion. First, each element is associated with specific emotions. Second, the theory defines how energy moves in the body. The third is how to manage the energy of the body. Let's look at Five Element theory to understand how to use nature and help with the stress of being a caregiver.

PART 4: The Emotional Challenges & Chinese Medicine

Sometimes I don't even know that you are gone...

-Kim

I don't know if caregivers think about the emotional challenges ahead. When I started out on my caregiving journey, the emotions I was going to experience were not even a thought. From the start, I was focused on the action "how-to" part of caregiving.

How to create a safe environment. How to incorporate a new member into the household. How to do end of life planning. How to, how to, how to… The emotions just showed up.

There were the emotions I expected, like love, joy, satisfaction, amusement. It was the emotions I wasn't expecting that took me by surprise. The negative emotions took me by surprise and created an internal dialogue causing the most stress.

The problem with negative emotions is you can't get away from yourself. If you are having a bad day at work, you can go home, quit, find a new job. If the freeway is a nightmare, you can decide not to drive, get an Uber, call a friend. The only person you can't get away from is yourself.

In caregiving, emotions can start to surface and take control of your internal dialogue. Within a short time, you might find you have a chorus going on your head that keeps you up at night. And when left to their own devices, emotions can really take you for a ride. They can mix in self-judgment and self-criticism, letting you mentally punish yourself for your feelings. Taking care of a family member can bring up issues from your childhood that you thought were long gone. The "should haves" start to show up.

A significant body of research exists examining the physical demands and long-term emotional strain of caregiving coupled with the health risks to the caregiver. Some of the research indicates that highly stressful caregiving roles can increase your risk of mortality by as much as 63%. [26][27] Wow, that's a lot. On a positive note, the research also suggested that learning successful coping skills can increase the resilience of the caregiver and their life expectancy.[28] Yup, the purpose

---

[26] Schulz, R., & Beach, S. R. (1999). Caregiving as a Risk Factor for Mortality. *Jama, 282*(23), 2215. doi: 10.1001/jama.282.23.2215

[27] Perkins, M., Howard, V. J., Wadley, V. G., Crowe, M., Safford, M. M., Haley, W. E., … Roth, D. L. (2012). Caregiving Strain and All-Cause Mortality: Evidence From the REGARDS Study. *The Journals of Gerontology Series B: Psychological Sciences and Social Sciences, 68*(4), 504–512. doi: 10.1093/geronb/gbs084

[28] Lewitus, G. M., & Schwartz, M. (2008). Behavioral immunization: immunity to self-antigens contributes to psychological stress resilience. *Molecular Psychiatry, 14*(5), 532–536. doi: 10.1038/mp.2008.103

of this book is to learn strong coping skills, enhance your resilience, and life expectancy!

Coping skills can come in so many forms. Just knowing about the potential for negative emotions can be a coping skill. Like driving a car around a hairpin turn, knowing the corner is there gives you time to prepare to slow. Accidents are accidents because you don't know they are there.

In this section, I focus on the emotions I didn't know were coming - the negative feelings. The positive emotions didn't cause stress. The negative emotions did. Along with being a negative emotion, their presence tended to compound any stress I was feeling. The negative emotions made everything so much worse.

I don't know what life has in store for me. I will probably find myself in another caregiver role in the future just based on the growing prevalence of caregiving in our society. I don't want another chance to work through negative emotions in a caregiver's role. I don't want to see if I'll get better the next time. If I find myself facing my own negative internal dialogue again, hopefully, I can quickly engage the skills I learned this time.

To forgive is to set a prisoner free and find out the prisoner is you.

L.B. Smedes

Through your time as a caregiver, you will experience so many emotions. One that can have a negative influence on your health can be guilt. There will be those things that you'll review in your head and say, "Oh, I should have done this." Or, "Oh, I know better than that." You will always be able to find a reason to criticize yourself. Even today, working with my clients who are caregivers and talking through some of the tough issues that come up with dying, they will always find something that they haven't done correctly. I have my own list of self-criticisms.

There are no perfect actions. You are watching over another person who has their own needs and desires. The best you can do is be there for them. You can't stop the aging process, and you can't stop the natural progression of life.

That doesn't mean you will be able to stop the feelings of guilt. That's o.k. When you find yourself in the throes of guilt, remember the definition of guilt is "the fact of having committed a specified or implied offense." You committed an act, not a crime.

Emotions: Anger and Resentment / Wood

For every minute you are angry, you lose 60 seconds of happiness.

Anger and resentment are two additional strong emotions. The role of the caregiver asks for long hours and is emotionally draining. Without caregiving, you drive to and from work in rush hour traffic, make meals, grocery shop, scheduling appoints, pay bills, coordinate activities, and on and on. Adding the role of caregiving means you do this for two people and have no time for yourself.

The person you are caregiving will have constant requests for your presence and assistance that may get overwhelming. If you are caregiving for an aging adult, every day, they lose more and more of their daily functions. You will need to help them accomplish more and more of their everyday life and tasks.

If you are raising your grandchildren, you will notice that you don't have the energy you had when your kids were young. Even though kids gain more independence as they age, the vibrancy and vitality of youth will exhaust you. It doesn't mean you love them less. It means you don't have the energy you once had, and exhaustion can impact your emotions in ways you might not want to think about.

Taking care of your spouse during or after a major illness can be personally devastating. Couples who have lived together for long periods have built a life together. Couples usually split up the tasks of the household. It takes the two of them to ensure a well-run home. When one of the partners gets ill, all the roles fall on the other spouse in addition to the caregiving role of nursing them back to health or just nursing them.

Being tired all the time and not having personal time, you will get frustrated. You can get angry and resentful. You might even say things you are going to regret later.

Caregiving is a role where you are better off if you learn self-forgiveness. You are doing the best you possibly can. Sometimes the best you possibly can isn't enough. That's o.k. You are going to up-end your whole life to become a caregiver. You are going to put your life on hold. You are going to lose personal time. All of this can create a pressure cooker.

So, you get angry, resentful, say something you'll regret later. Is that the worse you could do? No, the worse would have been leaving them to their own devices and homelessness.

When anger, resentment, frustration gets the best of you, take a minute to acknowledge you are not proud of what happened because that makes you human. Take a moment to think about what you could do differently. Maybe there is something. Perhaps there isn't. If you ended up saying something you regret, apologize. Tell them you are sorry. If it makes sense, explain what you were feeling and how their actions were impacting your life. Their actions may have threatened something like safety or respect or understanding. An excellent framework to help put these conversations in a positive light is Marshall B. Rosenberg Non-Violent Communication.

The person you are taking care of might not even understand what you are talking about. But it makes you a better person.

Emotions: Fear / Water

One of the best tools to help manage fear is to implement a process - a step by step process.

-Kim

Fear is the one insidious emotion. You don't even know fear is there or fear is driving you to respond and act in weird ways. Fear lays low and can feel like nervousness at times. Because fear is about perceived threats to your safety and security, the standard defense mechanism to fear is the need to fight and protect yourself or run and save yourself.

At times your response to fear can be anger. You angrily defend yourself to protect ourselves. Most of the time there are no reasons for the anger. For some, the response to fear is avoidance. You don't talk about issues and pretend the problems don't exist. Some of us respond to fear with fear, an uncomfortable sensation of foreboding.

Because fear can cloak itself in so many different garments, it may take a bit of time before you can really identify fear driving your emotions.

Fear has as its trigger safety and security issues. If someone is talking to you about a bill and you find yourself suddenly angry, a financial security issue could have been triggered. If you are experiencing financial strain, finding another expense usually doesn't help.

For me, it was a financial issue. I didn't budget finances but was always on top of them. With my mother, our expenses took a significant increase due to travel costs, transportation costs, managing multiple households, remodeling the house to accommodate her, etc. etc.

There were so many expenses I couldn't keep a grip on them. And then my husband and I had some personal financial catastrophes which just sent the finances into a tailspin. I was panicked. I felt like our financial security was at risk, and I couldn't see an end.

One of the best tools to help manage fear is to implement a process - a step by step process. It takes the focus off the problem and towards a solution. I applied a personal budget capturing all the miscellaneous expenses swirling around the house and entered them into the budget. I added in our income and started monitoring the outlays. When I watched the budget, I was able to find a solution and realized we were still afloat, and it was o.k.

Fear likes a process. A process is like walking yourself off the ledge. If it is a safety issue, identify the safety issue, and start brainstorming solutions. Pick the best solution or the best solution for your situation and figure out the implementation plan. Then do it.

Here is another example some of you may be facing. My mother wanted to live on her own. Both my husband and I thought living on her own was a safety issue. We brainstormed how we could make safer living independently. Technology became a big part of the solution. Camera technology took a leading role. We researched and tested the available technology, identified which worked in a manner acceptable to us, and implemented the winners.

We had a three-step process. The first step was to identify what we needed in camera technology. We needed a live and remote monitored video with storage. That meant we needed to have an internet solution. We needed a useable resolution of 1080P. The solution had to be dependable. Dependable was a 99% uptime and the ability to reconnect to the internet if the cameras experienced an error. We needed night vision. We needed the solution to record only when sensing movement because we didn't want to go through hours of useless video. Voice was nice to have. Notification of movement was a nice to have, and we didn't need remote police calling.

The second step was identifying the cameras, and the third step was testing them. Based on our criteria, we tested four different systems: Swann wired system, Ring, Canary, and Yi.

The wired system was truly cumbersome, and video quality was crappy. I never got to the remote monitoring part as it just got too tiring after wiring the cameras and viewing the monitor. The storage was local and had to be cleared out when full. It was challenging to figure out if anything happened since it was just an endless stream of video. There were absolutely no bells and whistles on the system. Bells and whistles would be two-way audio or remote notification. The technology was just so dated it was a waste of time.

Next, we tried the Ring. The system is reliable, about 95% of the time, and can take good quality pictures. If it disconnects, it automatically reconnects itself. All the cameras had two-way audio, night vision, and remote notification of movement. These systems worked great outdoors. We ended up keeping the Ring system outdoors but balked at the price to add internal home cameras.

Because the Canary was getting so much coverage, we thought we would try the camera. The system only works about 65% of the time. It disconnects itself a lot and needs manual intervention to get back online. Sometimes reconnecting can be a long process.

Since we were doing this for a senior, a senior usually can't reset the system. The picture quality was crap. But it did have two-way audio and was the only system that could monitor air quality and home temperature. By setting the sensor to "Away" mode, it would video capture movement, which is what we wanted. The annual monitoring fee was expensive, especially if you were using more than one camera and especially since it was down so much of the time.

The last camera we tried was on a whim based on a tech blog. I was starting to feel the financial pinch of camera technology and was a little hesitant to try the Yi cameras. Yet, nothing we tried was really working indoors. The Yi cameras were inexpensive, at times, being only 1/3rd the cost of the other cameras.

Wow! The cameras were cheap, flexible, easy to set-up, had two-way audio, remote monitoring, video storage either local or on the cloud, good picture quality, and were up 100% of the time – seriously, 100% of the time. But then they had added features of pan and tilt, motion tracking, and cheap annual video storage options.

After we had identified and tested the cameras, the ranking was easy. The Yi cameras won hands down, and I haven't regretted that decision since. Out of all the technology we implemented, the cameras were the most valuable and significant investment. They significantly helped with the fear of my mother's safety and helped manage my worry.

Fear- identify the issue, pick a process, and do it. Our fear issue was safety, we identified a potential solution through cameras and implemented a test and selection strategy, and then we did it.

Issue: Safety

Potential Solution: Use camera technology to reduce safety concerns

Cameras:

- Swann wired system
- Ring
- Canary
- Yi

Criteria Must Haves:

- Internet solution
- Smart phone access
- Live and remote viewing

- Video Storage

- Automatic reconnect if disconnected

- Resolution equal or greater to 1080P

- Record only when sensing movement

- Uptime of 99%

- Set-up is understandable and low maintenance

Test Cameras and rate the cameras against the criteria. Note any nice to haves which may influence the decision.

Emotion: Grief – Metal

When I watch the rain, I realize that even the world cries. Yet, after the storm is when genuinely amazing things can happen.

-Kim

There is nothing I can say about grief. Grief happens in so many ways and so many different times. The big thing about grief is grief is the emotional response to a loss that identifies you. Whether it is the loss of a relationship or the loss of your old life, these losses helped identify what made you and created your life. Losing any of it is like having the leg of a stool kicked out.

Grief isn't learning to live without. It's that you learn to rebuild that leg and go on. In the meantime, while you're still working on rebuilding your stool...there is grief. For that, I have found no better partner to help me walk through grief than Chinese Medicine.

Grief likes time. It wants to be by itself. The problem with grief is it is painful. Not only is grief painful, but it also cannot be hurried. So, for something that is painful and doesn't like to be rushed, grief can last for a long time. Avoidance becomes a significant way to deal with grief.

The most common method of dealing with grief I have seen in my practice is by being busy. You're running, running, running all the time doing much more than you are physically capable of. You can't rest because the minute you slow down, the grief becomes much more prominent. Pushing yourself to be busy when you're already exhausted can create more issues. Your patience can get shorter, your flashpoint comes faster, excessive exhaustion can lead to anxiety in Chinese Medicine. The anxiety turns into panic attacks.

When I watch the rain, I realize that even the world cries. Yet, after the storm is when genuinely amazing things can happen.

Emotion: Anxiety - Fire

Anxiety is so much more than just another emotion.

-Kim

Anxiety is the most disturbing of all the emotions. I had never experienced anxiety until I became a caregiver. Before my personal experience with anxiety, I considered anxiety another feeling equal to all the other emotions. What I learned is anxiety is so much more than just another emotion.

Anxiety is pervasive. It is the most internally damaging. Anxiety just hangs out at a low level and sometimes at a high level. Anxiety likes to be there all the time. It is there when you are sitting down watching television, waking up, or trying to go to sleep.

Chinese Medicine can help explain why anxiety is so severe. Anxiety can be an emotion of the heart channel. The heart has the responsibility to incorporate and create meaning of all the feelings we experience.

The emotions involved in caregiving are centered around love. They deal with our connections, closeness, and compassion. In caregiving, we come face to face with the loss of someone we love. Maybe we won't lose them today or tomorrow. But, in the back of your mind, you know you will be saying good-bye sooner than later.

Saying good-bye doesn't even have to be their passing away. Saying good-bye can be forgetting your memories of being together. Saying good-bye can be changes in their personality, inability to communicate, forgetting daily activities. Saying good-bye could be your grandchild growing up or your spouse, parents, grandparents succumbing to the disease.

Caregiving comes at you from all angles.

· There are increased physical demands.

· There are increased mental demands as you start incorporating the mental juggling of another's life.

· There are the emotional demands that being a caregiver brings up.

And all these demands hit you at once. You usually have the emotional stability to integrate one of these items into your life. But caregiving requests you blend all these items at the same time. Over time, the pressure of having to manage all the aspects of caregiving starts to exceed our ability to cope or integrate.

Any powerful situation that exceeds our ability to cope or integrate is going to create anxiety inside us.

The definition of trauma is a profoundly depressing or disturbing experience – a powerful emotional experience. Most of us can deal with one trauma. If the wounds are well spaced with the time between them, we can deal with many injuries in life. In fact, we do deal with many traumas throughout our lives. Where caregiving can be different is the lack of time between events and the length of time spent in caregiving. Many caregivers are spending multiple years caregiving without a break. At some point, their reserves are going to be exhausted. They will no longer be able to integrate all the emotions. That is when the caregiver begins to experience anxiety.

When anxiety first hit me, I wasn't sure what was happening. I just knew that I was super uncomfortable. The anxiety felt like a nervousness with no direction. Anything could trigger it. By the end of being a caregiver, even small events could start an internal dialogue of nervousness.

What really surprised me was that my symptoms fit the description for PTSD. I was dealing with anxiety that was happening with even small issues. Something would happen, and I would just start fixating on it. I would blow it up in my head, making it bigger and bigger, and I couldn't stop. I couldn't sleep. I couldn't sit still.

What I didn't know when I started out on this journey is that PTSD can happen after any traumatic event. PTSD doesn't have to happen immediately. You can think you have your personal life altogether. You can believe you have found the right coping skills, and one day it just goes sideways. The clue that there was a potential for PTSD was coping skills.

It is estimated that 7 or 8 out of 100 people will experience PTSD at some time in their life[29].

To be diagnosed with PTSD, you must be diagnosed with events in each of the following four categories that have lasted more than a month and affect your daily activities. If the symptoms go away in a month, it is considered Acute Stress Disorder (ASD).

1. At least one re-experiencing symptom that can be flashbacks, bad dreams, or frightening thoughts.

---

[29] National Center for PTSD. (2018, September 26). Retrieved from https://www.ptsd.va.gov/public/PTSD-overview/basics/how-common-is-ptsd.asp

2. At least one avoidance symptom can include staying away from places, objects, or events that remind you of the experience or avoiding thoughts or feelings related to the event.

3. At least two arousal and reactivity symptoms that include: being easily startled, being tense or "on edge," difficulty sleeping, angry outbursts.

4. At least two cognition and mood symptoms can include trouble remember critical features of the event, negative thoughts about yourself or the world, distorted feelings of guilt or blame, and loss of interest in enjoyable activities.

Anxiety is the same as and a little different than all the other negative emotions. It is the same as the other negative emotions because it affects one of the key elements in Chinese Medicine and can be treated with Chinese Medicine. It is different because the element is fire.

Chinese Medicine states the responsibility of integrating all the emotions from the other elements falls on fire. Fire takes the emotional input from the different elements and applies meaning. Meaning incorporates and creates understanding and direction.

I was angry because my favorite shirt was ruined. I was sad because I lost my charm bracelet. I was afraid because I heard a weird sound. Fire is the element that adds the "because" to your emotions. Without the "because," you become a jumble of emotions running around in your head without meaning. You don't know why you are sad. You don't why you are angry. You don't see why you are fearful. Without the ability to apply meaning to emotion, our emotions become confusing and disorienting. They seem to stay in your head because the only way to get them out is through using a "because" statement with them.

In Chinese Medicine, the lack of a "because" statement means you can't integrate your experiences into your psyche. In Western Medicine, the most common time you see the inability to incorporate lessons into the mind is with post-traumatic stress disorder.

Fire enables us to take emotion and discern meaning. The other elements are blinded by their desires and will seek their longings with no remorse. It is fire that must translate the desires through a filter of conscious, intelligent thought called discernment. Fire takes the emotions and can go further than just applying meaning to feeling, fire can allow you to change your response. Fire will enable you to change your interpretation. Fire can allow you to change your behavior.

Fire's responsibility starts to highlight why anxiety can be such a painful emotion to overcome. Anxiety can be challenging because it is more than just one feeling. It is your interpretation of your world, and that interpretation has gone off track due to the overwhelming amount of emotional stimulus.

Anxiety begins to help you see how carefully crafted your world is. Your emotional responses are consistent and predictable. But add in caregiving, and as the stress starts to increase, the variance in emotional responses begin to grow. As the emotional highway starts to get burdened with more and more emotional traffic enters, traffic jams appear. More accidents happen. Driving becomes more complicated as more drivers enter the freeway.

This is anxiety.

Even after your role of caregiver has ended, the emotional highway will still be at full throttle. It takes a planned, collaborative effort between you and your psyche to find an exit and stay off the road.

Emotion: Love - Fire

This is your own private journey into yourself, and for the person you love.

-Kim

I've spent all the time talking about the negative side of the emotions. For each element, there are also positive emotions. I want to take just a minute to swing back to why we started on this journey of caregiving in the first place.

For the fire element, the positive emotion is love, the integration of all feelings. Love is the reason you took on this role. Love is the reason that you are committed. Love is why whenever a negative emotion comes up, the negative emotion is so confusing.

I have never heard anyone regret their commitment to caregiving. I've listened to a lot of people regret not participating, but I've never heard of anyone regretting their commitment. No matter how hard it was, how painful, how much trauma came forth.

The further away from the end, the more people rejoice they were there in the end.

Wherever you come in the spectrum of caregiving, caregiving is started from your depth of love. After it is over, love will be there in the end. How you handle yourself during the caregiving part will determine how hard the aftermath will be.

Caregiving is also the time where you re-avow your ability to love selfishly. All the positive aspects of love can come to the forefront with caregiving. You learn how to be unconditional. You learn how to be protective without being overbearing. You learn how to be accepting without giving direction. You learn patience to allow everyone to find their own way.

And each one of these items is about learning about yourself.

The only thing I know for sure is all healing comes from unconditional love. This journey is about being the best you can be. It is not about being perfect. It is not about what others think you should feel or do.

This is your own private journey into yourself, and for the person you love. Protect your journey.

PART 5: Listening to the Elements

I'm finally ready to write about this.

-Kim

It took a long time to get to this part of my story. Even today, as I stare at my computer screen wondering about time, I have no idea. Part of me wonders if it was something as simple as wanting to find the most effective way to explain some of these concepts. The topic is so vast and can be viewed from so many different angles. Whatever I write here would only be an eyedropper of information. I worry that it will not be enough or make any sense.

I can feel the imbalance in my Earth element as I overthink my solution.

Here is my attempt to explain Five Elements.

In Classical Chinese Medicine, there are five elements. The elements are the root. A statement I read has vast meaning. Yet, even the initiates say without the proper education, it means pretty much nothing. I can understand what they meant because it would be like me looking at Newton's Law of gravity in 900 BC and trying to understand the vast meaning behind a small formula. The statement was:

"The five elements are before, during, and after. They were the first, and all life comes from them."

In Chinese Medical school and many of the introductory books on five elements, the five elements are taught as a "noun." A noun describes an object...something we can touch and hold. This works well in a western thought process. If an object can be seen, it can be defined. The ability to see an object supports the belief the elements are a thing limited by boundaries.

But five elements are not a thing. They are an allegory of life that describes energy and movement. Learning nouns does not teach what the elements represent. For me, the original classroom teachings of five elements as a noun was actually detrimental to my ability to practice the medicine effectively.

With the elements, their true meaning has nothing to do with being an element, a season, an emotion. All these things are an outline. The true nature of the five elements is movement. All life starts with movement...a heartbeat, a breath, the energy of the sun, the coolness of the moon, the pull of gravity, the big bang theory. Therefore, the movement was at the beginning. Movement is here today in the middle. And movement or the lack of movement will be at the end.

Finally, the statement made sense. Movement is energy. There can be no movement without energy. Surprisingly enough, there is a set of rules or principles governing the conduct of movement.

To get a feel for how essential the principles are - the earth spins in one direction. The sun rises in the east and sets in the west, and that is the rule. In the west, the governing principle is defined by physics and force, which has our planet in motion, and motion will not cease until an opposing force changes the action. If for some reason, you woke up with the sun rising in the west, you would know there was a problem.

The guiding principles of movement are the guiding principles of energy. You know the heat of the sun must give way to the cool of night, or the earth would burn up. Life can't be sustained if only one type of energy is present. If it was always night, life would perish.

The five elements explain the different types of energy and movement. The elements include guiding principles to better understand how movement and energy interact with each other.

The spinning of the earth changes day to night

and night to day. The spinning of the planet also brings about changes in the seasons. In each season, the overall energy is different. Yet, each season is vital for life. To miss or eliminate a season would terminate life. An imbalance in any one season will have far-reaching effects on all subsequent seasons.

Part 6 has an actual example from nature. You can read how changes to the late run salmon slowly deteriorate the health of the surrounding areas over subsequent years.

Chinese medicine sees the elements in everything and are the building blocks of you. The elements are in everything because every microcosm is a smaller expression of the macrocosm. The elements are defined to help give guidance and direction. They can show how to interact with the world. They can help identify where mental, emotional, spiritual, and physical support is needed. By learning about the elements, you learn about yourself.

The first appearance of elements in Chinese Medicine is not clearly dated. It could be 5,000 years ago, it could be longer, it could be shorter. For sure, the teaching was consolidated during the Han dynasty between 200 AD and 200 BC. The elements were grouped into what is called the Five Element Theory.

Well, enough of history.

The elements outline the natural progression of life. Life is represented as a never-ending circle. Movement and time start at any point on the ring. Maybe it starts with the harvest in the fall. Or, the patience and regeneration of winter. Or the birth of spring, the fulfillment of summer, or the transition of seasons. Life can start anywhere on a circle that only moves in one direction. Winter can not go back to fall. The elderly will not grow-up to be younger. Movement will always follow a route called forward.

Much of what is taught about the elements is based on the seasons and the experience of each season. To better understand the elements, watch nature, watch the changes of the seasons, watch the interaction of life through a season. You don't need a guru or me to better understand the elements. Yet, a guru or me can share different perspectives, which can help you see various aspects of the elements.

The elements consolidate information from the seasons and become more than a season. They become a personality with emotions, preferences, opinions. They have a combination of characteristics that form a distinctive character. In the world, they are components that make up the planet: water, wood, fire, earth, minerals. In the person, they are ruled by officials masquerading as yin organs.

In ancient China, the emperor had vital officials responsible for the critical roles of the government. The positions were determined to be mandatory to a well-run government. The officials had specific strengths needed for their job.

In Chinese Medicine the body is viewed as a government with key officials. The officials are the five yin organs: heart, spleen, lung, kidney, and liver. Each one of the yin organs has a role as the ambassador to an element in the body.

Each person has every element within them. They say in Chinese Medicine, every person will favor one element over the others. Even though everyone has all the elements, each individual prefers one of them. And two of them are usually the core of the personality.

Here are the five elements, their organ, and their official role.

Eleme	Orga	Official

Fire	Hear	Emperor/Sover
Earth	Sple	Storage Official
Metal	Lung	Principle
Water	Kidn	Health Official
Wood	Liver	General

The next chapters will introduce the elements and the emotions associated with the element. Each section will discuss the emotional best and worst of each element.

The chapters will help you understand how energy moves through the elements. You can use this information to understand how an element out of balance can impact another element and how one element can be balanced by another element.

Then you will get to see how to pick the right element to help release your stress and give you a quick pick up to allow you to continue your journey as a caregiver.

Water: The Health Minister/Self

None of us want to be In calm waters all our lives

-Jane Austen

Water has unique properties. The most interesting is that ice floats instead of sinking in water. The solid form is lighter than the liquid form. The heat capacity or amount of heat needed to increase the temperature of water by 1 degree is more than twice rock and minerals. Water is the vital substance that allows our planet to remain temperate because it can absorb so much more energy/heat than solids. More solids dissolve in water than any other material.

I mention this because it is a unique feature of water. A core strength of water. Water's ability to keep the earth temperate…Water can make sure that things don't get too hot and that temperatures stay moderate and comfortable. This core strength of water is expressed in a well-balanced water person.

My husband is a water person. I've watched him time and time again diffuse frustrating situations with a gentle, disarming sense of humor, and patience. Water is patient. Long after I know my head would explode, my husband is still looking at the problem, trying different angles, and listening to different solutions.

Water is comfortable, likes to be secure. Think of being in a pool of water and hold your breath under water. There is a gentle, nurturing comfort that can be found in water.

Water can feel heavy and slow. Water is not in a hurry to get somewhere. In fact, it really doesn't like to set a direction. Water likes going with the flow and is good at it. Water is cooling just as it cools the temperature of the earth, it can cool and hold the energy of the body. Water is Yin.

What water needs is patience. Water shines as a role model. Much that drives them directs them to be a role model. They want others to acknowledge them for their ability to set an example. They want to set an example. Water is a gentle, compassionate nature which can make them a great role model.

The energy of water is the essence of life. The two kidneys represent heaven and earth. The core foundation of our human existence is rooted in water.

When water is under pressure, things change. The temperature of water goes up as the molecules start to move faster and faster. Water expresses this discomfort as fear. Fear is a healthy emotion and can keep you safe. The goal of fear is to move back to safety and comfort – the province of water. Fear can become a negative emotion if it becomes a constant companion.

Fear can be expressed as avoidance. Avoidance is the most common pathological emotional expression from unbalanced kidney energy. The desire for safety and comfort drives the water energy to quickly move around and avoid the problematic situation… all difficult situations…even those that have small impacts.

Ice, a whole lake that moves freely in the summer, becomes frozen and immobile in the winter. Water can be stubborn and absolutely refuse to move. When the stubbornness becomes severe, out of balance water stops seeing the situation around them and makes assumptions on what is happening. They close their eyes and plant their feet. The stubbornness is no longer reasonable and is based on an internal dialogue that has nothing to do with reality.

Wood: The General

Werifesteria: to wander longingly through the forest in search of mystery.

Wood is represented by spring. The energy of spring moves upward and out. The season of spring utilizes a considerable amount of energy in birth and growth. It is the time when plants spring forth and reach upwards. Spring movement makes growth and expansion a key theme for the Wood element.

Wood is lively and full of hope. Spring is the season of hope for a good harvest, to find a mate, for a good year. Wood expresses the ability to hope.

There is a lightness and rapidness to the Wood element. Spring is about constant motion with purpose and direction. The seed always moves towards the sun even when planted upside down. Animals always move towards reproduction.

Wood is goal-oriented, and goals need plans. That means Wood is a good planner. Wood will naturally be able to put together thoughtful ideas and detail potential alternatives. They excel at strategy and can vision long-term.

The Wood person is thoughtful and kind. Their personality and force are powerful, like the trunk of a tree. The tree can withstand the force of storms and still stand. Yet, like a tree, Wood is flexible, having the ability to sway in the wind and grow around obstacles.

Justice is also a need for the Wood element. Justice is an opinion about how we administer fairness. There can be many different opinions on equity and justice. Justice can be based on principles of equality where every person has equal benefit. Or, our democracy indicates that all persons have a right to a fair say in society. Or justice can encompass the legal obligations of government. Justice entails thousands of different thoughts. The Wood person will have a clear idea of justice for them and tend to stay true to their beliefs.

Yet, when the wood energy in the body is out of balance, there are several different ways unbalanced Wood shows up. The ability to maintain constant motion through the Wood element can be misused. Probably the most interesting way in which it appears is through distracting ourselves by always staying busy. When dealing with a situation that causes deep unrest, a simple way to avoid the situation is by staying active.

Caregiving is one situation that can cause deep unrest. Caregiving creates all the emotions, including fear, grief, anger, hurt. The easiest way to not deal with any of these emotions is by staying busy.

There is a strong force in the energy of spring. Life springs forth, and when blocked, the emotional expression is anger, frustration, and resentment. There is so much energy being blocked, and the force of it continues to build up. When the power becomes too strong to hold back, the heat breaks through as explosive anger. Like a vent tube that blows off the excess steam, anger explodes in flash and then disappears.

Yet, another way to look at Wood is in the boards of Wood we use every day to build homes, furniture, etc. Boards are rigid. Out of balanced Wood can have rigid thoughts, be demanding, inflexible, judgmental.

Fire: The Emperor/Sovereign

The most wasted of all days is the one without laughter.

E.E. Cummings

The element of Fire is associated with Summer. Maybe today, when you hear the word "fire," you imagine the worse of it. You see more about the wildfires ravaging the landscape or global warming overheating the planet. Yet, thirty years ago, that was not the case. When you heard the word "fire," thoughts of a relaxing campfire on a fall evening shared with family and friends roasting marshmallows and eating smores came to mind.

When I think of summer, I can see the last warm days of summer and fun nights canoeing on the lake or basking on the beach. I feel the hot summer sun on my skin and light clothes - activity and comfort.

Or, farming comes to mind and how summer finishes the crops. How crops can take everything that came before and integrate it into the best plant possible. Here we see all the hopes of the spring planting coming to fruition.

The element of Fire and the season of summer can be open, joyful, relaxed, and able to integrate everything into one thing.

In your body, the fire element applies meaning to emotion so you can incorporate the feelings into your psyche and everyday life. Just like crops integrate everything from the environment to become the best crop possible, the fire element integrates all your daily emotions to become the best potential for you.

Some years, farms get too much rain. Crops can't integrate all the water. Some plants fail, some crops are stunted, some crops are affected for a while, and then recover. When we get bombarded with emotions, the fire element can get overwhelmed and is no longer able to incorporate our feelings and reactions into our psyche. Like flooding, we start to get overwhelmed with trying to find meaning and acceptance in our actions and the actions of others around us.

One of the toughest things about caregiving is emotions. Loving the person we are taking care of sometimes is not enough to avoid negative emotions.

Then there is the person you are taking care of who is going through their own internal struggle. Their struggle can make your whole interaction so much more difficult. They can be going through depression, resentment, unacceptance, dementia, distrust, grief, fear....

For myself, as a caregiver of an aging parent, the amount of internal conflict was magnified when my parent began to express exhaustion with living. Just coming to grips with their desire to stop living was incredibly unbalancing.

Similar issues happen with a partner or spouse. One of the complexities of aging will be experiencing a significant medical concern like dementia. It isn't just all the household tasks you've picked up. You have all the tasks and have many things you didn't have before. Suddenly, you must be constantly vigilant and own complete management of the house. You might experience loss of friends, loss of your best friend even though they are still here, daily grief over all the losses, and all the other things that come with caregiving. All these things can make it difficult to remember the good.

Being overwhelmed can create resentment, fear, anxiety and a host of other negative emotions. Because you're overwhelmed, finding time to sort through a gallon jug of uncomfortable feelings can be a little daunting.

The most common emotion tied to an overwhelmed fire element is being flooded with a sense of nervous tension with no identifiable source. Almost anything can trigger it. You find you can't stop thinking. Your thinking may not be directed at anything.

As the fire element gets more and more out of balance, the nervousness can start to feel like jumpiness. You begin to create drama in your head. You find yourself obsessing over little details that have no real meaning. You blow-up these details making them bigger than mountains.

Other emotions can start to marry with nervous anxiety. You may begin blaming yourself for some of your actions because, in retrospect, you didn't think you handled a situation well. Criticizing your efforts opens the mind to believing other people may be criticizing you. This internal criticism can breed distrust of those around you and can make you defensive with others.

It all starts with trying to come to grips with emotions that arise in caregiving.

What starts out as nervous energy grows into jumpiness, anxiety. Your sleep may be impacted. You might find yourself crying over nothing and unable to stop yourself. You can't turn off your brain and have a hard time concentrating. Your nervousness creates incessant chatter in your head or with others. You may have heart palpations, panic attacks, or a feeling of foreboding that has no discernible source. An unbalanced fire element is super uncomfortable.

Earth: The Storage Official

Life tried to crush her but only succeeded in creating a diamond.

-John Mark Green

Earth, I think this is the best element of them all. This, of course, is my bias. Yet, Earth is the center of it all. When we think of the Earth, we have a tendency to think of the planet we live on. The stable and constant nature of the ground represents vital aspects of Earth. Earth is calm and grounded. Also, a balanced Earth is level-headed and focused.

Other aspects of an Earth person are the concept of being content and stable. All these characteristics tend to make an Earth person easy to be around.

Earth is noted for protecting and storing things of values. Part of the function of the storage official is to keep track and oversight of objects kept in storage. In charge of protecting what is valuable, their ability as an administrator comes to the front. Another title given the element of Earth in ancient China was the Administrator of Granaries. They were responsible for organizing, protecting, distributing, and counting grain inventories.

They needed to ensure processes were in place to safeguard the stocks. Today, I tend to think of accounting when I consider the responsibilities of Earth.

The balanced Earth person, besides being level-headed and grounded, tends to be stable and content. They can stay grounded even under stress. With their desire to organize and supervise, the Earth person can be a beneficial resource.

When the element of Earth gets out of balance, the first indication can be obsessive thinking. Problems become an excellent source for the mind to begin endlessly thinking about. The inability to stop thinking about the problem makes it difficult to go to sleep. Waking up in the middle of the night and starting right back in on the issue is another sign.

Obsessive thinking usually takes on the costume of problem-solving in your personal life. It can be something as simple as, "Did I lock the door?" Or it can take on that self-judgmental tone of, "I should have done that better, how could I miss that...."? The problem can show as compulsive or repetitive chatter with themselves or with characters they have created.

Obsessive thoughts can devolve into jealousy. Jealousy crops up when your self-judgment becomes too much, and you look to ways to avoid yourself. Seeing other people, you imagine they have beautiful lives without self-judgment.

This can lead to selfishness. Selfishness is about being concerned excessively or exclusively for oneself. The concept of obsessive thinking that is focused on oneself can be further expanded to conceit or excessive pride in oneself. Other terms include vanity, narcissism, or egotism. Self-admiration can fall into this category.

I had a horse. My horse was always such a ham, and I found him so entertaining. Being that I ride in arenas with mirrors, he had this habit of having to watch himself in the mirrors. He was very enamored with himself. We would come off a line of jumps heading to the mirrors, and he would get distracted having to check himself out in the mirrors and making sure he looked his best. He was the apex of self-admiration. He was so funny.

It wasn't until later through a blood test that I found out he had a sugar problem like diabetes. In Chinese Medicine, the spleen and stomach, the earth element, are critical players involved in diabetes. Disease in Chinese Medicine must go through many layers, including the mental and emotional layers before becoming physical.

The emotional aspect of Earth out of balance is the feeling obsession. It can devolve into jealousy, selfishness, conceit, arrogance. When this element is out of balance, your tendency is to be harsh with yourself and with others.

Metal: The Principle Official/Prime Minister

We begin to remember not just that you died, but that you lived...And that your life gave us memories too beautiful to forget.

I think the role of the caregiver is embodied in the energy of Metal. The Metal element is associated with Fall and all that comes with the season of harvest.

Not many decades ago, most of the population lived on the farm. Although that demographic has reversed itself with 95% of the people living in the cities, we still associate Fall with a harvest. The trees prepare themselves for winter. The leaves turn yellow, red, brown, and fall to the ground. The fields are harvested, left barren with the stubble of the year's harvest. The weather loses its warmth, and a cool, crispness begins to encroach on the days and nights.

There are a few themes that permeate Fall. One is exhaustion, another is death, and the last is the bounty. The warmth of summer activity has exhausted the plants and animals. Now, they prepare to bed down for the winter. Leaves and crops have come to fruition, and their life is coming to an end.

There is slow patience to fall. It doesn't happen immediately. The changes come first in the rising and setting sun. The light becomes softer as the sun changes its trajectory across the earth's sky. The days begin to shorten. The weather follows as a coolness starts to invade our days. The trees slow down and begin to store their nutrients deep inside for the winter. The leaves fall. The fields stand dry and ready for harvest.

Fall is a time for a significant change, a reversal of energy. From the vibrant push forward, the energy now turns inward and becomes quiet, reflective. The energy has changed from yang to yin. Conservation, retention, preservation becomes significant themes. These themes are very different from Spring, where exploration, extension, discovery are the key themes. Or the energy of Summer where fruition, relaxation, growth, maturation are themes.

The change in energy is a reversal making the Metal element and Fall a transition period in life. As with all transitions, transitions come with change. The Metal element becomes a significant transition in life. It is a time for letting go and starting a new challenge. Metal no longer is trying to create the world. Metal gets to experience the world. Metal can sit down and experience the world, which makes the time of Metal a time to be accommodating. This can be a time of great generosity. Here is the time when many people feel the push to give back.

Fall is a time when all the presumptions of the prior seasons are emptied and no longer hold the relevance they once did. We are no longer so serious. Fall is a time when one is more inclined to be open and honest, making us more accessible to others.

Coping and accepting change becomes a new life lesson. Done well, there is an openness and willingness to accommodate. There is a joyousness with people and with life. Sometimes I think of this as the "Best is yet to come."

The best can be seen in the harvest of your life. In this harvest, you can find great joy or great sorrow. Both emotions help define the energy of Fall.

When this energy is out of balance, a person will feel excessive sadness and grief. This is the time of harvest. Not only do you get to reap your life's work, but you also get to let go of many of your relationships, activities, etc. Friends and relatives start to pass. Things you could do when you were younger are no longer feasible. Health concerns crop up. Life and death issues come much closer.

The letting go can become disorienting and leave you feeling unbalanced. The relationships and activities that use to define you might suddenly disappear. Surprisingly, your life is defined by your relationships and activities. Losing these definitions can leave a sense of disorientation. It can make you question your existence, leaving you feeling unbalanced or lost.

For me, the unbalanced Metal energy is most clearly expressed in the "mid-life crisis." I had thought the mid-life crisis was something I would never feel. When I was growing up, the label was a negative label tacked on men who abandoned their responsibilities at a time when it was least expected – at the end of it all.

What I came to find out was a mid-life crisis was created out of loss. When the losses were too much and overwhelmed your coping skills or your ability to accept and accommodate the change, or the grief and regret played such a substantial part in your lives then a mid-life crisis had fertile ground to pop up.

The mid-life crisis was not anything that I thought it was. It was something so much more visceral and human. It came out of a desire to slip back into the past, back into a time when everything was still o.k. A desire to be back where people, youth, endless possibilities still were in front of you instead of behind you.

When Metal gets significantly out of balance, the questions change to, "What is the point?" or "Why am I here?" Things like a loss of direction can leave us confused and disoriented. Our instinct is to swim back to the known shore. You want to be in familiar surroundings, familiar dreams, expected life outcomes.

The only thing that exists is the here and now. The out of balance Metal energy takes time to process the grief and sadness, and it is going to take the time it is going to take. It always takes much longer than expected.

For me, both the balanced and the unbalanced Metal energy highlighted a big part of my caregiver role. The much more profound meaning came in the end because the end came on so fast. I had been at the apex of being overwhelmed. I was running my business. I was trying to manage my mother's life. At the same time, she was living long-distance (completely impossible). I was flying weekly to my sister's bedside and trying to finalize last wishes. Then it all just suddenly ended. This cacophony of noise suddenly came crashing down into silence.

The silence was deafening.

My sister left. A month later, my mother left. A month after that, my horse went. For my whole life, these relationships had defined me. Their life applied their energetics to my life. Their presence was intricately intertwined in my own being. Suddenly they vanished.

It was as if some amazing magic trick had happened, and with the touch of a wand, the stage was empty. I stood alone in the center of a darkened stage under white light in utter silence. All the activity that preceded was gone and no longer was there any distractions to hide the force of Metal with its grief, pain, and sadness.

I found myself in the middle of a mid-life crisis. I found myself going back to places from my past, almost as if trying to find them. All the while, I was dragging behind me quiet despair, knowing they were no longer there. Knowing I could no longer reach out touch and talk to my family.

PART 6: How Energy Flows

The sky would be awfully dark with just one star.

Chinese Medicine looks to our universe to understand how energy flows. The belief is that everything in the world is inter-related. Everything in the universe is connected and influences the other. Fundamentally, it makes sense. In fact, you would have to be inter-related with the rest of the world, or else you would be dead. Right? You would be on the wrong planet trying to survive in an environment where your existence was not part of the DNA of the earth.

You can look at the living matter and see it is made up of carbon, oxygen, nitrogen, hydrogen, and phosphorus. The closer you get, at the molecular level, the more all life looks the same. The further away you get, like in a plane 30,000 feet over the planet, all life appears the same. There is a tiny area of space where you can create boundaries and divisions to identify separate individuals.

Chinese Medicine used this inter-relatedness of things to examine and make hypotheses about the human body. One aspect of Chinese Medicine concerns how energy moves in the body. The movements were identified as cycles. Probably the most well-known flow of energy is the supporting cycle. Seasons are used to help understand the cycles and energy flow. In the West, you usually start with spring, which relaxes into summer. Summer slows down to fall, which sleeps in winter.

Four primary seasons. Yet, in Chinese Medicine, there are five elements. In the Five Element Theory, the fifth element is rectified by the creation of a fifth season called late summer. Late summer falls between summer and fall. And who knows, maybe in ancient China there really was late summer. And perhaps time and distance have forgotten this season. Yet, maybe not entirely. I remember growing up being grateful for a season you called "Indian Summer." Indian Summer was an extension of summer, where you were able to enjoy the warmth of summer just a little longer.

You know the seasons can only move in one direction – forward. Winter can never come after spring. Just as fall can never come before summer. Each season has a time and place, and everything must come in its time and place to survive.

I love that...time and place... There are such patience and acceptance to that very statement. I grew up in the West and learned little reverence for time and place. Here, in the West, speed and gratification were the key drivers of my early years. Maybe, as I grow older, I see the need for time and place.

You can look at nature to understand why the ancient Chinese understood the concept of time and place. You've heard many examples of how life is changing patterns, and these changes have far-reaching effects.

I live in the Pacific Northwest, and salmon is a part of the Northwest. Over the past decade, more and more research has gone into studying an abnormal phenomenon where the late-run sockeye salmon are coming in earlier and earlier. Sometimes, the late summer run is coming in at the same time as the summer run sockeye salmon.

The research is showing that over 90% of the late-run sockeye salmon are dying before laying their eggs. Before 1995, when the late run came in at its proper time, late run salmon mortality rates rarely exceeded 20%[30]. Time and place.

So, seasons have a time and place. And everything within the season has a time and place. Keeping time and place ensures balance and health.

If the fish do appear at their proper time, their role in the food web stays intact. If they don't show up at the appropriate time, the loss of over 90% of the run reduces the population for the subsequent years.

The impact of this keystone species on the environment is impressive. In Alaska, salmon contribute almost 25% of the nitrogen in trees resulting in trees that are three times taller than areas without salmon[31].

---

[30] Cooke, S. J., Hinch, S. G., Farrell, A. P., Lapointe, M. F., Jones, S. R. M., Macdonald, J. S., ... Kraak, G. V. D. (2004). Abnormal Migration Timing and High en route Mortality of Sockeye Salmon in the Fraser River, British Columbia. *Fisheries, 29*(2), 22–33. doi: 10.1577/1548-8446(2004)29[22:amtahe]2.0.co;2

Another interesting fact is salmon contribute phosphorus to the surrounding vegetation. Phosphorus is necessary for photosynthesis and is used in fertilizer. It is estimated a good salmon run in the Lake Iliamna area of western Alaska can deposit 170 tons of phosphorus.[32]

So, the late run coming in at the wrong time has an impact on the size of the sockeye population. The change will magnify over the years. Nature can survive one insult, just like our body can survive one abuse.

Reviewing the impact of sockeye salmon on the environment and studying the gradual decline in sockeye salmon population helps me better understand a term commonly heard in Chinese Medicine, "engender."

Each season engenders the subsequent season. So, late summer engenders fall. When the season of late

---

[31] substancedev, A. (n.d.). Why Protect Salmon. Retrieved from https://www.wildsalmoncenter.org/work/why-protect-salmon/

[32] Willson, M., Martson, B. H., & Gende, S. (1998). Fishes and the forest, Expanding perspectives on fish – wildlife interactions. *Bioscience, 48*(6). doi: 10.2307/1313243

summer is healthy, late summer can lay the groundwork for the following seasons to flourish. Whatever is created in its season is the foundation for the all the future or all of life. I say all of life because the current season is the foundation for every future event. The strength of the current season determines the energy that can be given to all future events.

Let's look at farming. A late-season freak hailstorm destroys the harvest. What is created in late summer lays the foundation for the next season. The fall harvest is reduced, which puts the foundation for the upcoming season. Winter sees much starvation and death. Although death places nutrients back into the soil for spring, the smaller population could harm the following season and take many years to recover.

What I've been talking about, the seasons, and their effect on the subsequent season is called the supporting cycle in Chinese Medicine. It is a theory of energy movement in the body. The model for the theory is a circle that reflects the seasons and the element for each season. In the model, the elements are the exact same size and take the exact same amount of space on the circle. The model emphasizes that each element is equally important. A weakness in one element will affect all elements.

The supporting cycle is described as a mother/child relationship. Summer is the mother of late summer, and late summer is the child of summer. Late summer is the mother of fall, and fall is the child late summer. In the supporting cycle, the child is the element that follows on the circle. The child is the subsequent season or element.

You say things like the mother nourishes and takes care of the child. You use examples of temperament to explain pathology like an unruly child exhausts the mother.

The mother and child relationship are true, but it tends to simplify our understanding of how significant each season and element is to the overall well-being of the environment. When you look at energy movement in the supporting cycle as a mother/child relationship, you fail to see the element after the child, which is why I started with the concept of engendering.

You can see the concept of "engender" when you look at the late summer salmon example. It is easier to understand the consequences of abnormalities in the sockeye salmon example. You can easily understand the mammals and birds that feed off the salmon eggs will have a much smaller harvest and face food constraints and starvation. The smaller sockeye salmon fish runs will bring fewer nutrients to the area the following year and reduce the health of the surrounding forests.

As time goes on, the gradual decline will have a larger and more significant impact on the environment surrounding the sockeye salmon run spawning areas. Let's say the late-run sockeye salmon disappear completely, and a third of what is left of our salmon population is a loss. The reduction in nutrients to the area will slowly begin to erode the health of the surrounding forests. Mammals and fowl depending on the late run to survive the harsh Alaska winters, will experience the loss of their primary food source and begin to die off. The surrounding forests will start to deteriorate, and the waterways will lose a key player in keeping the streams and trees healthy.

I talk about this because my family has been struck with cancer. The mother/child relationship is a valid way to look at the movement of energy in the body. Yet when you need to make major changes in your life, the analogy is oversimplified.

Engender is the ability of nature to accept insults until it can't. It's the same with energy movement and health in the body. The body can take many insults. The body takes years of partying, years of staying up late studying, working odd hours and multiple jobs, eating on the go and fast food, years of a stationary lifestyle. The body can do this until it can't. There will be many warning signs along the way. Do you listen and try to change how you manage our body, or do you forge fearlessly ahead, ignoring the warning signs of your body?

Each element lays the foundation to create the next and subsequent element. What happens in an element is not limited to the element or the following element. What happens will impact all of life. Each element is part of an interwoven web where one movement moves the whole network.

Most of the time, you forge fearlessly ahead – myself included. You have done these things for so many years, they have become an aspect of your identity. Each insult has a ripple effect that moves like a wave through the whole body. So, when it comes to things like cancer, the wave has become chaotic. To calm the chaos, every aspect of your life may need to be addressed.

Most of us are aware of the yin and yang in Chinese Medicine. You have seen the circle with a white and black part called a taijitu. Part of what the taijitu symbolizes is the transformation of yin into yang and yang into yin. What was once yin will transform into yang and what was once yang will transform into yin.

The concept is most easily expressed by the imagery of day and night. Day turns to night and night turns into day. In all experience, you have not known day or night to exist without the other. If day or night were to exist without the other, everything would be dead because life needs both daylight and darkness to survive. Life needs movement, and when day or night exists without the other, movement has ended. As a living organism, the only way you are alive is through movement, movement of our heart, our lungs, metabolic movement.

When movement stops, you cease to exist. Just as the only way day and night can exist without each other is when the earth stops spinning. The earth would have to become a solitary meteor floating stationary in space with the light constantly shining on one side and darkness on the other. Only at that point, when earth floats silently through space, no longer spinning, will yin and yang cease to exist.

But, you say, one side is light, and the other is dark. How can yin and yang cease to exist because the earth has stopped spinning on its axis? Yin and yang are not about light and dark. Yin and yang are about movement. Yin and yang are about the energy of motion. Light and dark are only symbols to help understand the waxing and waning of movement. Light and dark are not the result. Movement is the result.

If you look at the four seasons (five if you look at ancient China and Five Element theory), each season is one part of a year or one piece of an annual life cycle. Each part of the life cycle has equal importance. Spring, summer are considered yang and makeup one side of the coin. Fall and winter are considered yin and make up the other side of the coin. Late summer sits on the cusp or the edge of the coin and is almost neutral.

Yang, the energy is more forceful and is full of movement. Yin, the energy begins to relax and regenerate. You need both. You can only have a great, active day if you have given yourself enough time to renew.

So, you have different seasons that go in a specific order. Each season is equally important and must complete the tasks of the season to give the appropriate energy to the subsequent season. Each season has a type of energy, which is either yin or yang, and describes the predominant tasks of the season. The tasks can only be completed successfully if the appropriate resources were gathered from the previous seasons.

That is the supporting cycle. The supporting cycle follows the order of the seasons. The energy goes from robust, to joyful and relaxed, the winding down, to regenerate. You can see the supporting cycle in something as simple as a day in our life. With a good night's sleep, you wake up refreshed and robust, ready to go. By afternoon, our energy is slowing down and starting to relax. As evening comes, you begin to wind down, watch a little TV, talk to family, read a book. And then it is time for bed where you fall asleep and regenerate.

A season engenders the following seasons. Whatever energy the season brings to the table is the energy that will support the coming season. The next season won't get any more or any better energy. What it gets is what it gets. Although you can correct one-time insults, chronic and long-term insults slowly start to take their toll on our body until you are sick with some disease.

Let's look at tasks not being completed well. You stay up late one night, but still must wake up early for work. You wake up tired and groggy and drink coffee to push your fatigued body to move forward. Most of the day is a push as you work to stay awake and complete tasks. Half-way through the day, the boss askes everyone to stay a couple hours overtime to finish an important project for a customer. When work finally ends, you are too tired to make dinner and swing by the fast food place to grab a burger which you eat on the way home. When you get back, you don't have time for the family or kids and immediately go upstairs and go to bed.

Sleeping through our "family time" allows us to catch up on our sleep and recover for the next day. Even though the family feels left out and forgotten for that evening, they recover and forgive your absence.

Yet, if this pattern becomes more chronic and long-term, catching up on our sleep becomes harder. Our mood starts to waiver. You become irritable. Our family sees less and less of us and begins to feel resentment about our absence. One insult, you can survive. Multiple, chronic insults start to leave a mark.

The other movement of energy in the body is the control cycle. Here, the elements are still on the same circle in the same order. In the control cycle, each element has the responsibility to control another element. On the ring, let's look at the fire element. The fire element skips the child element, earth, and controls the subsequent element, metal. And it goes like that for each of the elements.

The symbolism of the control cycle is rather straight forward. Fire melts metal. Earth dams' water. Metal cuts wood. Water drowns fire. Wood binds earth.

If you look at it, control is the power to influence or direct behavior or the course of events. I like to mix Western and Eastern medical concepts whenever I can. Here, the control cycle is very much like the concept of homeostasis in Western Medicine. The control cycle is there to adjust and try to keep things in balance.

Just like homeostasis in Western Medicine, the control cycle is a response to a change in the internal environment.

Unlike Western Medicine where medications are used to alter the internal chemistry of the body, Chinese Medicine uses the concept of energy flow to help strengthen weak areas to bring the body back to normal function.

So, Fire (summer) controls Metal (fall). One way to look at the control cycle is to use the analogy of Fire melts Metal. Let's say you make steel and find that your steel has a weakness due to improper formulation. You may be able to melt the steel down and reformulate to correct the formula.

That is not such a good analogy. Let's look at it from the emotions. You know each element is associated with an emotion. Where Fire is associated with summer and summer is a time to relax and enjoy, the emotion associated with summer is joy. Metal is associated with fall and the harvest and dying of things. Metal is associated with grief.

When the emotion associated with the element of Metal, grief, gets out of control, look to the controlling cycle, Fire, to bring the element back into balance. Fire is associated with the emotion of joy. So, in Five Element Theory, a method to bring grief back into balance is laughter. That makes sense. If I'm sad, go find something funny to watch on streaming or sit and watch kittens or puppies playing. Just thinking about sitting down to kittens or puppies playing picks up my mood. Do you ever wonder why there are so many videos on YouTube about kittens and puppies being cute? Well, now you know.

These are two models of energy movement that will help you bring yourself back into balance as you live through the ups and downs of being a caregiver.

PART 7: Nature and the Elements

You are the universe expressing yourself as a human for a little while.

-Eckhart Tolle

Ancient China saw five elements in the world. It was believed to, we had to have these five elements. We didn't need them in equal amounts. We just needed some of each. The five elements are Fire, Earth, Metal, Water, Wood.

Each of the elements brings its energy to the table. To better understand the energy the element brings, Chinese Medicine uses analogies with things in nature to help explain and clarify the energy the element brings to the table.

The Fire element is most commonly associated with fire, and can also be associated with the sun. Fire is a yang element. Yang elements lack substance – they are more ephemeral. Fire also has many expressions, from cozy to inferno. Yet, each of the expressions is imbued with heat and warmth. For comfort, the warm, cozy glow of a campfire is brought to mind. For wrath, the infernos are represented in some of the wildfires and deliver a different heat.

The earth element is represented by earth, the soil, the land. The ground can be the rich, fertile lands of the Midwest or the sand of the Yuma desert. In each of these soils, a different type of environment is supported. Earth is more substantial or physical and is considered yin.

The Metal element can be represented by minerals, rocks, and the sky or air. The Metal element is represented by the lungs, which have the responsibility of exchanging gases in the body. The Metal element is the change from yang energy to yin energy. It sits on the cusp or the edge. If you look at a coin, you have heads and tails, and in between the two is the cusp or edge of the coin. This marks a change in direction. Daylight is changing to midnight.

The Water element is represented by water from rain, to creeks, to rivers, lakes, and oceans. Water makes up a large percent of our body and our planet. The Water element is cold and the most yin of the elements.

The last element is Wood, represented by Wood. Trees, plants, shrubs all take on the essence of Wood and show different aspects of Wood. From a Doug Fir, which can grow over 200 feet and live longer than a thousand years, to the grasses on the plains which last only a season. The Wood element is the change of yin energy to yang energy. This marks a shift in the direction like midnight marking the change to daylight.

In nature, each of these elements has it's time. By participating in order and correctly, all life can continue to exist. Each of the elements is responsible for its energy and effort. Changing the energetics, the timing, or the length will cause significant changes and potential harm to future seasons.

Look to nature to understand the role of inappropriate action out of season. Long springs with late Mayfly hatches mean the Mayfly is not available at the appropriate time to nourish fish and the subsequent season. Our previous example of the slowly disappearing late summer salmon shows the missing run fails to feed the wildlife for winter and the landscape for the next season.

I always think of cancer as the most perfect example of a system pushed out of balance to such an extent that the system must perish. Breast cancer is a perfect example. In Chinese Medicine, the liver channel usually plays a role in breast cancer.

The liver organ and channel are partnered with the gall bladder organ and channel. The gallbladder channel travels along the side of the body and the breasts. Have your acupuncturist needle gall bladder 22 or 23 and feel the relief that comes from those points to get a feel for just how much energy is traveling along the channel and getting stuck in and around the breast area.

In Chinese Medicine, disease usually comes from the Dao to the spirit to the emotions to thoughts to the physical body. The feelings associated with out of balance liver is anger, frustration, repressed anger, explosive temper, judgment, controlling attitudes. Many of the clients I have treated with breast cancer have repressed anger and frustration. The energy it has taken to contain their resentment takes a tremendous toll on their body. Fatigue and exhaustion are common feelings that cause depression.

The most common expression of depression is exhaustion or the inability to do anything. Everything sounds like so much effort. Even if you only have one thing to do, the one thing can feel overwhelming.

And frustration, resentment, anger at some point, and time usually need you to decide to change something. These are usually big changes. They are not something as simple as changing clothes. They are something as complicated and scary as looking into yourself and accepting yourself. That glimpse within can cause a tsunami within your current life.

Everyone has a tsunami which needs to be faced if you are to change your world for the better. Sometimes it is accepting there are some things you cannot change. Sometimes it is accepting that you need to change. Sometimes...sometimes...sometimes...

In the breast cancer example, the decision to change is not made. For whatever reason...fear, selfishness, anger, anxiety, self-doubt, self-esteem, rigidity, self-worth, safety, desire...Whatever the reason, the decision is not made. More energy gets stuck in this gall bladder channel.

Any energy that is stuck doesn't move. A bruise is an example of fluids getting stuck. Over time, most bruises go away as the body can manufacture enough immune system elements to repair the damage. Yet, sometimes we suffer a trauma the body can't fix completely. Scars from surgery, car accidents, lipomas, and other such traumas can be too big for the body to repair back to perfect condition.

In Chinese Medicine, energy that gets stuck for too long begins to create phlegm and then things like cysts, fibroids, lumps, etc. form. Chinese Medicine states cancer always comes from phlegm or the blocking of energy movement in the body.

To reverse phlegm, nodules, fibroids take a considerable amount of effort. Yet, in this example, one of the key goals would be to move the energy that is blocked in the gall bladder and liver channel.

In the previous chapter on energy movement, fire follows Wood in the supporting cycle. To help drain the excess energy of Wood stuck in the breast channel, stimulate the Fire channel. Laughter is the emotion of fire, and excess laughter can help drain the liver and gall bladder channel. Long walks on hot summer days can help drain the wood channel.

We hear it a lot with cancer…just go off and do what you have always wanted to do or do what you love. People can be healed of disease, doing what they love, and finding joy and laughter in life. Chinese Medicine theory tells us why laughter and joy can improve health.

This leads us to our last step, putting it all together.

PART 8: Putting It All Together

If your path is more difficult, it is because your calling is higher.

The last step is to take everything you have learned and put it all together. Putting it all together comes in 4 simple steps.

The first step is to identify your emotions. Even though it seems like an easy task, sometimes the job of recognizing our emotions is more complicated. The task can be complicated because we are complicated. There can be many layers to our feelings, making it difficult to truly pinpoint the actual emotion. We may be using one type of energy, like Spring and the liver, to avoid facing our real feelings. Or, the energy of Earth and the Spleen could be blocked by an excess in the Metal/Lungs. This can happen because of grief over the loss of someone profound like a child or a parent.

Yet, the task could be complicated because we use different words to express our emotions. The most common example is those emotional expressions that fall under the umbrella of anxiety in Chinese Medicine.

Anxiety can be a heart/spleen thing in Chinese Medicine. When it is a heart/spleen thing, the anxiety is the heart and spleen channel out of balance and usually a bit exhausted. The channels are exhausted because it took a long time to get to anxiety.

When I ask someone if they feel anxiety half the time, they will say no. But, if I ask if their thoughts are incessant and non-stop making it challenging to sleep, they will respond yes. If I ask if they feel an underlying nervousness that doesn't go away, they will say yes. If I ask if they feel a foreboding with no known source, they will say yes. If I ask if their hands sweat uncontrollably, they may respond yes. These are signs of imbalance in the heart and spleen channel and fall under the umbrella of "anxiety."

Maybe we don't like the term anxiety. We are not "anxious". We handle our life just fine. We are not that person with "anxiety." The term seems to be considered a sign of weakness instead of a common imbalance occurring due to years and years of dealing with life.

A reason identifying your emotions may be difficult is because you may not like the terminology. As you move forward with determining how you can use nature to help rebalance yourself, choose the option that has the most words which sound like your feelings or emotions. If it doesn't quite work out, try the next opportunity.

The two cycles of energy movement can help bring yourself back into balance as you live through the ups and downs of being a caregiver. The two cycles are the supporting and control cycle.

Process

The overall process is only four steps.

Step 1:

In step one, you identify your emotions. Identifying our emotions can be complicated because sometimes we have more than one feeling competing for our attention. Or, how we define an emotion uses different words. Or, we are not aware that we are distracting ourselves to avoid our true feelings.

So, don't get too wrapped up in perfecting your emotional identification. Just check those that you feel are most accurate and go from there. This is not an exercise in perfection. This is an exercise about life. If you get it entirely right the first time, then great.

You might also find that you already know which nature brings you the most amount of peace at this very moment. Sometimes, it is helpful to look at this process in reverse to identify the underlying emotions that are driving your need to be in that nature.

When I was caregiving, I was being assaulted from many different directions. I had really lost my balance in life and could no longer identify what I was feeling. I had an idea where I needed to go. What I found was a need for immense water and immense sky. The sky starts to talk to energy of Metal and lungs and grief. There was so much going on. The overwhelming amount of grief I was feeling was drowning by all the other emotions. This exercise in reverse helped me acknowledge how profoundly sad and lost I really was.

Who has time for any emotion when you are a caregiver...right? Yet, just acknowledging the feelings of sadness, grief, loss helped me come to grips and stay on track.

So, look at the toolset section and pick those emotions which best fit you at this moment. If you think you know where you need to be, use this process in reverse to identify your internal dialogue.

Step 2

The second step will help identify where you may find the most amount of support in nature. In Part 6, you read about two different cycles on how energy flows. The supporting and controlling cycle. Both cycles help pull you back into emotional balance.

The supporting cycle helps with putting things back into balance due to having too much energy in the channel or too little energy in the channel.

When you have too much energy in one of the channels, you can use the supporting cycle to help rebalance yourself. The supporting cycle states you can use the child to drain the excess energy of the channel.

I've written a lot about the liver channel. With so much familiarity with the liver channel, I'll continue with that example. So, let's say you have a lot of frustration and resentment going on. Almost overwhelming, something always ticks you off. In the supporting cycle, the liver is represented by Wood, and the next organ and element is the heart and fire. The emotions of laughter are bathed in sunshine and ripened fields, tall grass, birds.

In this example, the supporting cycle states use the child (fire/heart) to drain the excess in the parent (wood/liver). When you think about it, children can be a great distraction. If you are caught in emotions of frustration, and suddenly your two-year-old starts doing something you find hilarious, your anger immediately disappears. That is the concept of using the child to drain the parent.

But let's say you are feeling overwhelmed and exhausted, pissed off or depressed. Now, when your two-year-old does something hilarious, which includes tipping over the water glass, it is no longer funny and feels more like more work and no breaks. Then go to the parent of the liver channel or the grandparent. That makes sense, too. When you're raising your children, how often to you take them to the grandparents so you can get a break.

When frustration is coupled with exhaustion, you can't go to the child to drain the channel. There is nothing in the channel. Instead, you must help fill the channel back up. In the supporting cycle, the parent to the liver channel is water, and being around bodies of water will help rebalance an out of balance liver channel. When out of balance coupled with exhaustion, go to the parent of channel out of balance.

The controlling cycle helps from another perspective. The role of the controlling cycle is to help keep a channel in balance. When we look at the liver channel, the controlling channel is the lung channel or the Metal element. To help keep the liver channel in balance, a strong lung channel is a must. Spending time looking at the sky and watching sunsets can be helpful.

Because being a caregiver is stressful, the liver channel is always impacted. Being a caregiver usually lasts a long time, and by the end of it, exhaustion sets in. We have used so much liver energy, the liver has drained the parent and overwhelmed the controlling channel.

In practice, I have found that I've consistently used formulas to strengthen the kidney/water and the lung/metal channels/elements. Based on what we just talked about, the water element is strengthened to support the liver channel, and the lung channel is enhanced to help keep the liver channel in balance.

These formulas would be represented by water and sky in nature.

Step 3

The third step is simple, find the nature you need in real life. Try to make it a quiet place. You don't have to go far. It can be in your back yard. A fountain for water. Laying in the grass and looking up to the sky for

Metal. Can you remember doing that as a kid and how relaxing it was? A sunny day for fire or a fire pit. Gardens for the earth. Trees and shrubs for Wood. All of this can be found in your backyard.

If you have the luck of time, go find it in the world. I needed BIG water and drove to the ocean. In the Pacific Northwest, we still have beaches without people and with beach grass. It was amazing.

The third step is easy. To find your nature.

Step 4

The last step is to just sit down and wait. You don't have to do any meditation stuff. Don't even close your eyes. Just sit down and watch. Plan to give yourself a half-hour. Don't worry if you can't turn the chatter in your head off. That isn't the goal. The goal is to just sit down and watch nature. Nature will do everything else on its own because nature is the best, most patient teacher.

Nature will help you turn off the chatter when you are ready. That might not be until years after your role of caregiver has ended. Sitting in the right Nature, Nature will slowly drain what is in excess and fill what is empty. You just must sit with her awhile.

By the time you stand-up to go back and face your responsibilities, you will find yourself feeling more at peace and better rested. If you think the same amount of agitation as when you started, you are in the wrong nature. Review your emotions and try a new selection. Or, just try different aspects of nature until you find the one that fits. There are only five of them. So, it isn't like it's going to take you a long time to roll through the five. But here is the thing. Many people are totally disconnected from the emotions and the body. Because they are disconnected, finding their feelings could be tough. Take this process in reverse, and when you locate your nature, review the emotions to get a better understanding of yourself.

I had an example just recently. I was feeling overwhelmed and exhausted and headed out to the river to unwind. I spent 5 hours on the river and couldn't relax for the life of me. I felt just as wound up and overwhelmed as when I started.

I had to swing by a friend's house, and we were going to take a walk in a Doug Fir woods next to the house. I was hoping the time by the water would unwind me from an exhausting week before I had to head over to my friend's house. I got to the house and was still wound up and feeling unfocused. We took a walk in the woods, and within 3 minutes, I completely relaxed.

I had just chosen the wrong nature. When I went back and looked at the toolset, I realized that my Earth element was the element that needed balancing. When I was in the thick of caregiving, I needed water and sky. Yet, now my caregiving was over, my Earth element was more out of balance. That made a lot of sense. Loosing such a big part of my family was and is very unbalancing and ungrounding.

Tools

The following chart identifies the element, when you have too much or too little of an element, and where to go in nature to get back in balance.

Use this chart to help identify which nature you can use. You can also use this chart to better understand the different movements of Qi in the body. Start with your emotion and review the section on the various movements of Qi. Review the nature to use and see what nature your elements fall under and how the emotion relates to the movement of Qi in the body. Chinese Medicine states cancer always comes from phlegm or the blocking of energy movement in the body.

To reverse phlegm, nodules, fibroids take a considerable amount of effort. Yet, in this example, one of the key goals would be to move the energy that is blocked in the gall bladder and liver channel.

In the previous chapter on energy movement, fire follows Wood in the supporting cycle. To help drain the excess energy of Wood stuck in the breast channel, stimulate the Fire channel. Laughter is the emotion of fire, and excess laughter can help drain the liver and gall bladder channel. Long walks on hot summer days can help drain the wood channel.

We hear it a lot with cancer...just go off and do what you have always wanted to do or do what you love. People can be healed of disease, doing what they love, and finding joy and laughter in life. Chinese Medicine theory tells us why laughter and joy can improve health.

This leads us to our last step, putting it all together.

Elem ent	Excess Too	Deficie nt	Nature for	Nature for

	much	Too little	Too much	Too little
Fire	Uncontrollable crying, inappropriate laughter, excessive dreaming, unable to complete a task, lack of enjoyment, unable to feel inspired	Feeling edgy and irritable, unable to sleep, unable to feel comfortable sitting, difficulty being quiet with yourself, can't stop your internal chatter, difficulty sleeping, nervousness	Open fields, grass, gardens, yards/yard work, working or sitting in the earth add in rain, lakes, rivers nearby	Forests, tress, grassy fields, fireplace, campfires, add in windy places
Earth	Feeling heavy,	Feeling unground	Open skies, clouds, wide	Gardening, activities

difficult
moving,
stubborn,
thoughts
are foggy,
depression
with
oversleepin
g, too tired
or
exhausted
to do
anything,
inability to
focus

ed,
Worry,
Inability
to stop
the
internal
chatter,
unable to
sleep,
feeling
out of
touch
with
reality or
disorient
ed,
brooding,
constantl
y
thinking
about
certain
events or
people,
hankerin
g for the
past,
obsessive

open spaces,
mountains,
can add in
trees,
shrubs

with earth,
walking
barefoot,
fields,
lawns, parks

		thoughts		
Metal	Worry, feeling blocked, things feel insurmountable, feeling lost, feeling alone, things seem too tough to overcome	Can't prioritize, feeling lost, feeling alone, tired, feel out of touch or disconnected, inability to let go of past, sadness, grief	Water, oceans, rivers, lakes, rain, fields just before harvest, campfires, fireplaces	Open skies, planted fields, grass fields, walking/standing barefoot on the ground
Water	Fear, stubborn, unproductive, content with status quo even if it is harmful, comfort is a driving	Lack of motivation, lack of will power, easily discouraged, depression,	Walk through the woods or trees, wind, gardening, gardens, parks, walking/standing barefoot on	Water: oceans, lakes, rivers, rain, puddles, open skies, wide open spaces, clouds

	force, lack of compassion	restless, difficulty concentrating	the ground	
Wood	Anger, irritability, resentment, rage, nightmares, inability to plan life, lack of direction, overwhelmed by feelings	Passive aggressive, jealousy, lack of courage, indecision, timidity, indifference	Campfires, fireplaces, warmth, fields before harvest, open skies, wide open spaces, mountains	Trees, forests, woods, water: oceans, lakes, rivers, rain, puddles

PART 9: Legal Issues of Caregiving for Seniors: Some of my learnings

If you find it in your heart to care for someone else, you will have succeeded.

-Maya Angelou

The last thing I had to learn about was some of the legal issues facing aging. The topic is so much bigger than this chapter. Yet, the chapter is a good start and highlights some of the mandatory items you will want before things get too far along when you can no longer get them.

This section is geared towards the discussion for seniors. This section only gives an idea of some of the legal and technical issues I ran into to. The section is not a comprehensive list of the legal and technical issues you will have to face.

With all the dramatic changes going on in our legal, healthcare, and insurance industry, the information here may no longer be relevant, and is only provided for informational purposes. The information is anecdotal based on my personal experiences, and everyone will have different experiences. Many of your experiences will not be covered here. And even those that are, the dialogue here is limited to my own personal experience. This information does not take the place of you doing your own research and talking to licensed professionals in the appropriate areas.

Mandatory Documents

There are three documents which would be best to obtain early in the process. If you don't have them and later determine you need them, your senior may not have the capacity to execute the documents and then their end of life care and lifestyle is left to the whim of the first agency quick enough and smart of enough to get control of their assets. The three documents are:

1. Power of Attorney,
2. Health Care Directive,
3. Will/Trust.

The Power of Attorney gives you the right to make financial decisions. The Power of Attorney is a written authorization to represent or act on another person's behalf. A limited Power of Attorney only allows you to act for a specific situation like selling or buying a house. Usually, you don't want a limited power of attorney for end of life issues because the issues are so vast.

The Health Care Directive is important. Power of Attorney gives you the ability to make financial decisions. The Health Care Directive clarifies the last health requests of an individual. Facilities need to honor the directive.

The last item is the will or trust. Many people pass without a will or trust which is fine if you are on state aid and have no assets. Yet, if you do have any assets, even if it is a small bank account, without the will or a spouse, obtain the assets can be very burdensome.

Like all the documents, state requirements vary. Some require notarization, some need to be witnessed. These documents can be used in other states. Mine were from Minnesota. Minnesota has strong requirements. Usually two witnesses, the parties to the document are additional signatures, and it must be notarized. Even if your state doesn't require that much verification, you might want to ask for it just in case you need to travel to another state. You never know what their rules are and unscrupulous can be a common term when it comes to seniors.

Why are these documents important? At some point many seniors are unable to make decisions for themselves. Without a Power of Attorney, it becomes a legal issue to pay for their care. Care facilities want to get paid. They will go to court to obtain the Power of Attorney to pay the medical costs. A care facility has different goals than the family or the patient. With the Power of Attorney, the care facility will also control what care, where they get care, and when they get care. If you want to move your senior, most times the care facility will not allow that.

The Health Care Directive is the request covering end of life care. Without a Health Care Directive health care is directed to maintain life. What I have found in my practice and with my own experience as a caregiver, there comes a time when the patient is done. They are ready to go, and living has become too painful for several reasons. The most common reason life has become too painful is their health has deteriorated to the point where it is too painful to stay alive. Many Health Care Directives will have a Do Not Resuscitate clause. Without the directive and the clause, our Western medicine can keep their heart beating for a very long time.

Usually, without the Power of Attorney and the Health Care Directive, the care facility gets complete control over how to care for the patient. I found that caring for seniors is big business. For some unscrupulous facilities, gaining legal custody of your senior allows them to care for them in any way they want and allows them to keep them alive way pass the time the senior wants to be here.

Even with these documents, care facilities will be unscrupulous. I had both these documents and my mother had a "Do Not Resuscitate". I had my mother at a facility, and I was in another state. For some reason, I had to fax her Health Care Directive four times to different areas of the facility. For some reason, sending it to the administrator wasn't enough. And even with sending the directive to each of these different areas, the facility still sent her to the hospital to be resuscitated.

The facility did not call me to tell me they had sent her to the hospital. Even though I had Power of Attorney, they made these decisions without me.

I had not had an issue with any other facility and her documents. Just this one "unscrupulous" facility. The administrator told me she could not honor the documents because Arizona law states the senior must complete this with their doctor and the doctor must sign-off that she is competent to make these decisions.

We were way past the point of her being competent enough to make these decisions. I would think sitting with an attorney and having two witnesses would be equal to sitting with a doctor.

I caught up with my mom in the hospital and talked the hospital through her documents. I faxed the documents to the hospital. They were great. I was able to talk with a Palliative Care Nurse who had no skin in the game and really worked to find the best solution for us. We were able to find another facility that was fantastic and took care of my mom as she had wanted.

From what I've learned, the hi-jacking of seniors and forcing them to stay alive can be very profitable for a facility. The best option for a care facility is to be able to gain Power of Attorney. When the Power of Attorney doesn't exist, a facility can move fast to gain control of the senior. I had to watch this with one of my friends. Neither one of us had any experience in caregiving. We didn't know what was going on.

She tried to get an attorney. Trying to find a good attorney takes some effort. It took me 4 tries to find a good attorney for my mother's stuff. The attorney my friend had was a little fluffy between the ears. Left to his own devices, the attorney would have inadvertently signed over the Power of Attorney.

The care facility my friend was dealing with had experience in gaining Power of Attorney. Two days before the court date, the Social Worker who was working at the care facility, called my friend and her attorney indicating the facility had requested an extension and the court date was postponed. In general, most of us are not attorneys and can be easily taken advantage of with misleading information.

My friend just had a bad feeling about the information the social worker shared and thought she would just show up anyways. Her attorney didn't show up. Do you know, the court date had not been postponed? My friend would have been a no show and would have lost the Power of Attorney. Slippery, slippery, slippery.

Because caregiving is not our business and we usually had to take on the role overnight with no previous experience; the learning curve is steep. Not all care facilities are like this one. I've run into more amazing facilities than crappy ones. But the bad facilities can make our journey treacherous. The three documents could save you a lot of pain.

Funeral Insurance Policy

There may come a time when you can no longer care for your loved one. If they are low income, and a lot of our seniors are, state aid is available. Even if they don't fall under the category of low income and have some assets, they may need state aid when their assets run out. Care homes are expensive.

If you think your senior will need state aid, you can talk to the care facility and they will help you complete the paperwork. The senior will have to liquidate all their assets. Yet, there are some things you can keep in order to pay for other expenses associated with end of life. One of them is a Funeral Insurance Policy.

Every state will have different things that you can pull out of the liquidation. At the time I wrote this, Washington State allowed the senior to withhold $20K for funeral expenses. This money never gets combined with the monies to pay for medical expenses.

Request Medical Records Early in the Process

Within a couple weeks of being in any new facility, request records. They are surprisingly difficult to get your hands on and come in unique shapes and forms. If you ask early and can go request in person, they can be easier to access. You can get denials for a lot of different reasons. You'll need these records in order to get any state benefits.

The records you get may be missing huge tracks of information or have discrepancies between pharmacy records and facility records. A whole lot goes on when you request records. So, do it early and do it often. You might not ever need them. But if you do, it's easier to have them before anything happens than trying to get them after something happens.

Rehabilitation vs. Palliative Care vs. Hospice

These are three different types of care and each has a different legal definition and different care options. The goal under each type of care is different and is covered differently by insurance.

Rehabilitation is to help a person get back to functioning.

Palliative care is provided during life-threatening illnesses. Palliative care provides relief from pain and other symptoms of the disease. Palliative care offers a support system to allow the patient to live actively. Besides enhancing the quality of life, palliative care can positively influence the course of the illness. This means that palliative care is used in conjunction with other therapies that prolong life. Antibiotics would be administered when a patient is on palliative care.

Hospice, although like palliative care, has one key difference. The key difference is that hospice offers no treatment to prolong life and is offered at end of life. Antibiotics would not be offered under hospice.

My sister had stage four breast cancer that wouldn't give up. When my sister and I first faced these decisions, we didn't understand any of it. I did the research and told her what I found out. I always saw my responsibility to her as a source of information and unconditional support.

It is almost as if you get sick and everyone takes ownership of your life in a pushy, unbiased way. No one takes time to ask her what she thought. And no one was taking the time to let her make her own decision - because we all wanted the best for her, and we all wanted her to live.

There was so much sharing done out of love and a desire for my sister to live. And my sister wanted to live. One of her most difficult decisions was to accept hospice. She completely understood that she had lost her fight against cancer.

We both knew we were done. I tried to help her take a shower and we had to get up the steps to the second floor. It took a half hour and took what little vitality she had left. We spent that afternoon laying on her bed, talking about her feelings. I wish I had done that more.

It went so fast after that. The day she accepted hospice was the last day for her to get out of bed. Within a week, she barely woke up. And then she was gone.

Even then, I didn't completely understand hospice. I was able to experience the decision tree one more time a month later with my mother. Through that process, I had better help with the decision-making choices and felt more prepared to make the decisions. A palliative nurse worked with me. I included my brother on the decisions. I felt that I had the correct medical information and we were able to assess the potential outcomes of each option against my mother's requests.

My mother's case was more complicated as it involved facilities, she was not at home, and my brother and I had to make the decision for her. The addition of different facilities made the decisions a little more complicated. Having to take ownership of the decision was the worse. Yet, the assistance I received from the hospital made me feel more comfortable with the decisions.

Health Insurance

This section is geared towards the discussion for seniors and their health insurance needs. This section is only to give you an idea of what was happening in health insurance when I was caregiving for my mother. With all the dramatic changes going on in the insurance industry, this information may no longer be relevant, and is only provided for informational purposes. This information does not take the place of you doing your own research and talking to a licensed professional trained in health insurance.

My mother was covered under Medicare. What I've found is that you can sign up for Medicare or Medicare Advantage.

The Medicare Advantage is less expensive and markets some bells and whistles which makes it sound like a plan that is equal to Medicare. It was through my clients that I found out the plans were different in the fine print. It was in some of the details where Medicare Advantage paid less. I had a patient in a care center recovering from a stroke and it was in some of the rehabilitation work where Medicare Advantage covered less.

Like everything, the differences between Medicare and Medicare Advantage were not easy to find and would have taken the effort of reading through their entire policy manuals before purchasing. The thing is, those manuals are never easily available before purchase. And saying the 200-page policy manual is available for you to read and takes care of the issue of transparency is nonsense. I would never have found the differences in rehabilitative care payments. As the consumer, you can't make an informed purchase due to the lack of transparency in the policies. For me, because of the lack of transparency, I would just go with the plain old Medicare policy.

Medicare has a coinsurance instead of a co-pay. Coinsurance differs from a copay in that coinsurance is a percentage of the bill while a copay is a flat fee you pay on all services. Office visits today are about $450.00. With a 20% coinsurance, your responsibility would be $90.00. Conversely, a copay is a flat fee like $35.00 an office visit. In general, copays are usually less costly to the subscriber.

Yet, a co-pay isn't a benefit if the policy pays for fewer services – services that you end up needing – and you must pay for those services out of pocket.

On a Medicare policy, you can purchase a Medigap supplement policy. The Medicare Advantage policy does not need a Medigap supplement. If you have the Medicare Advantage plan, you cannot be sold a Medigap supplement. Medicare.gov has a good description of the Medigap policies.

The Medigap plans supplement the coverage of the original Medicare policy. What this means is the Medigap plans pay all or part of the coinsurance the subscriber is obligated to pay...the 20% coinsurance.

"All Medigap policies must follow federal and state laws designed to protect you, and policies must be clearly identified as 'Medicare Supplement Insurance'. Medigap insurance companies in most states can only sell you a 'standardized' Medigap policy identified by letters A through N. Each standardized Medigap policy must offer the same basic benefits, no matter which insurance company sells it. So, all Medigap A policies offer the exact same benefits, all Medigap B policies offer the exact same benefits and each state will have the exact same number of different Medigap policies available.

Cost is usually the only difference between Medigap policies. Not only will the cost of the policy be different on each policy A-N offered by an insurance company, the costs between insurance may be different for each policy. That means that Insurance Company 1 is offering Medigap policies. They must offer all the federally mandated Medigap policies. Each of the different Medigap policies will have a different price based on the benefits they offer. Insurance Company 1 and Insurance Company 2 both offer all the Medigap policies. The actual price for the Medigap policies can differ between the companies. Insurance Company 1 may offer Medigap A for $45.00 a month and Insurance Company 2 may offer Medigap A for $38.00 a month.

Within the plans A through N, plans E, H, I, and J are no longer sold. If you already had plan E, H, or I, you can keep them. Plans D and G have different benefits if purchased before 2010 versus after 2010. So, that leaves A-D, F, G, J-N.

The Medigap plans usually vary by your out-of-pocket costs. You must look at each of the plans offered in your state. On each plan, you are responsible for the Medicare deductible of $185.00. When I was looking at the plans, Medigap B had the best coverage paying the full 20% coinsurance on Medicare Part B, a $0.00 hospital admittance fee on Medicare Part A, and a $0.00 Medigap deductible. Medigap Plan F covers the same as Medigap Plan B after you pay a $2,300 deductible on the Medigap plan and, when I was looking at them, the cost was about ½ of Medigap B.

Other plans have you cover 0%, 5%, 10% of your coinsurance and can include a fee for each hospital admittance. Those admittance fees can be high ranging from around $350 to around $1,400. When someone is nearing end of life, it is not unusual to get admitted to hospital about every two weeks for the last four to six months of life. In addition, some of these supplements will have a Medigap deductible that can range from around $2,300 - $5,500.

The more you pay for your medical care in coinsurance, deductibles, and admittance fees, the cheaper your Gap plan will be. The difference between Medigap Plan B versus Medigap Plan F can be about 50%.

A Medigap Plan is not mandatory. But, to survive the financial hit of a major health incidence, they are.

The supplemental must be purchased before a couple medical situations happen including the senior being diagnosed with dementia.

Lastly, today you can find a supplemental that covers Acupuncture and Chiropractic.

PART 10: In the End

Somewhere on your journey, don't forget to turn around and enjoy the view.

In the end, more and more are becoming caregivers. More people are finding themselves taking care of family members, friends, and even strangers.

The care giving population is growing, and it is expensive to be a caregiver. I've heard from more caregivers who had to take a person into their home. The financial cost was unexpected and, at times, risked their financial stability.

The stress of the becoming a full-time caregiver takes a toll on health, marriage, family, and friends.

Becoming a caregiver was probably the most difficult thing I've done, and I wouldn't have given it up for the world. This was a personal journey for me. It was my opportunity to support and give to my loved ones in a way that would never have been asked.

There is a raw honesty that comes with being a caregiver. It is a position that will define you. Daily, I was confronted with myself and my decisions. I was challenged to define my sense of right and wrong. I was pushed to become a better person.

I would have preferred to not have gone through this experience because then the people I loved would still be here. Yet, it was so important for me to be there for them. It was the one way I could tell them how much I loved them.

I wish you great insight, peace, and happiness on your own personal journey as a caregiver. I wish you the resilience and vitality to manage your life as a caregiver.

Appendix A: Stages of Dementia | Symptoms & Progression

There are several different scales which help you understand the progression of dementia in caregiving for the elderly. The GDS or Global Deterioration Scale for Assessment of the Primary Degenerative Dementia I really like because it gives timeframes. Everything about caregiving is about knowledge. The more you know, the better you will be able to navigate the waters.

The following information was found on Dementia Care Central at https://www.dementiacarecentral.com/aboutdementia/facts/stages/. This is a well-organized website that was funded by National Institute on Aging. It provides information, education, and support tools for caregivers.

Global Deterioration Scale for Assessment of Primary Degenerative Dementia (GDS)

The most common scale is often referred to simply as GDS or by its more formal name the Reisberg Scale. The GDS divides the disease process into seven stages based on the amount of cognitive decline. This test is most relevant for people who have Alzheimer's disease, since some other types of dementia (i.e. frontotemporal dementia) do not always include memory loss.

(Reisberg, et al., 1982; DeLeon and Reisberg, 1999)

Diagnosis	Stage	Signs and Symptoms
No Dementia	Stage 1: No Cognitive Decline	In this stage the person functions normally, has no memory loss, and is mentally healthy. People with NO dementia would be in Stage 1.
No	Stage 2:	This stage is used to

Dementia	Very Mild Cognitive Decline	describe normal forgetfulness associated with aging; for example, forgetfulness of names and where familiar objects were left. Symptoms are not evident to loved ones or the physician.
No Dementia	Stage 3: Mild Cognitive Decline	This stage includes increased forgetfulness, slight difficulty concentrating, decreased work performance. People may get lost more often or have difficulty finding the right words. At this stage, a person's loved ones will notice a cognitive decline. Average duration: 7 years before onset of dementia

| Early stage | Stage 4: Moderate Cognitive Decline | This stage includes difficulty concentrating, decreased memory of recent events, and difficulties managing finances or traveling alone to new locations. People have trouble completing complex tasks efficiently or accurately and may be in denial about their symptoms. They may also start withdrawing from family or friends, because socialization becomes difficult. At this stage a physician can detect clear cognitive problems during a patient interview and exam. Average duration: 2 years |

| Mid-Stage | Stage 5: Moderately Severe Cognitive Decline | People in this stage have major memory deficiencies and need some assistance to complete their daily activities (dressing, bathing, preparing meals). Memory loss is more prominent and may include major relevant aspects of current lives; for example, people may not remember their address or phone number and may not know the time or day or where they are. Average duration: 1.5 years |
| Mid-Stage | Stage 6: Severe Cognitive Decline (Middle | People in Stage 6 require extensive assistance to carry out daily activities. They start to forget names of close family members and have little memory of |

Dementia)	recent events. Many people can remember only some details of earlier life. They also have difficulty counting down from 10 and finishing tasks. Incontinence (loss of bladder or bowel control) is a problem in this stage. Ability to speak declines. Personality changes, such as delusions (believing something to be true that is not), compulsions (repeating a simple behavior, such as cleaning), or anxiety and agitation may occur. Average duration: 2.5 years
Late-stage	Stage 7: Very	People in this stage have essentially no ability to

Stage	Severe Cognitive Decline (Late Dementia)	speak or communicate. They require assistance with most activities (e.g., using the toilet, eating). They often lose psychomotor skills, for example, the ability to walk. Average duration: 2.5 years

Functional Assessment Staging (FAST)

The second scale is called the Functional Assessment Staging Test or by the acronym FAST. FAST also employs a seven-stage system based on level of functioning and daily activities. However, FAST focuses more on an individual's level of functioning and activities of daily living versus cognitive decline. Note: A person may be at a different stage cognitively (GDS stage) and functionally (FAST stage).

Functional Assessment Staging (FAST)

Stage 1 — Normal adult
No functional decline

Stage 2 — Normal older adult
Personal awareness of some functional decline.

Stage 3 — Early Alzheimer's disease
Noticeable deficits in demanding job situations.

Functional Assessment Staging (FAST)

211

Stage 4 — Mild Alzheimer's
Requires assistance in complicated tasks such as handling finances, planning parties, etc.

Stage 5 — Moderate Alzheimer's
Requires assistance in choosing proper attire.

Stage 6 — Moderately severe Alzheimer's
Requires assistance dressing, bathing, and toileting. Experiences urinary and fecal incontinence.

Stage 7 — Severe Alzheimer's
Speech ability declines to about a half-dozen intelligible words. Progressive loss of abilities to walk, sit up, smile, and hold head up. (Reisberg, et al., 1988)

Clinical Dementia Rating (CDR)

The Clinical Dementia Rating (CDR) scale uses a five-stage system based on cognitive (thinking) abilities and the individual's ability to function. This scale is more commonly used in dementia research and less so as a communication tool between medical professionals and patients and their families. This is the most widely used staging system in dementia research. Here, the person with suspected dementia is evaluated by a health professional in six areas: memory, orientation, judgment and problem solving, community affairs, home and hobbies, and personal care and one of five possible stages is assigned.

Clinical Dementia Rating (CDR) Scale

CDR-0 — No dementia

CDR-0.5 — Mild
Memory problems are slight but consistent; some difficulties with time and problem solving; daily life slightly impaired

Clinical Dementia Rating (CDR) Scale

213

CDR-1 Mild

Memory loss moderate, especially for recent events, and interferes with daily activities. Moderate difficulty with solving problems; cannot function independently at community affairs; difficulty with daily activities and hobbies, especially complex ones.

CDR-2 — Moderate

More profound memory loss, only retaining highly learned material; disoriented with respect to time and place; lacking good judgment and difficulty handling problems; little or no independent function at home; can only do simple chores and has few interests.

CDR-3 — Severe

Severe memory loss; not oriented with respect to time or place; no judgment or problem solving abilities; cannot participate in community affairs outside the home; requires help with all tasks of daily living and requires help with most personal care. Often incontinent.

View References

de Leon MJ and Reisberg B. An Atlas of Alzheimer's Disease. The Encyclopedia of Visual Medicine Series. Parthenon Publishing, Carnforth, 1999. Available at: http://www.alzinfo.org/clinical-stages-of-alzheimers

Reisberg B et al. The Global Deterioration Scale for Assessment of Primary Degenerative Dementia. *American Journal of Psychiatry.* 1982;139(9):1136-1139.

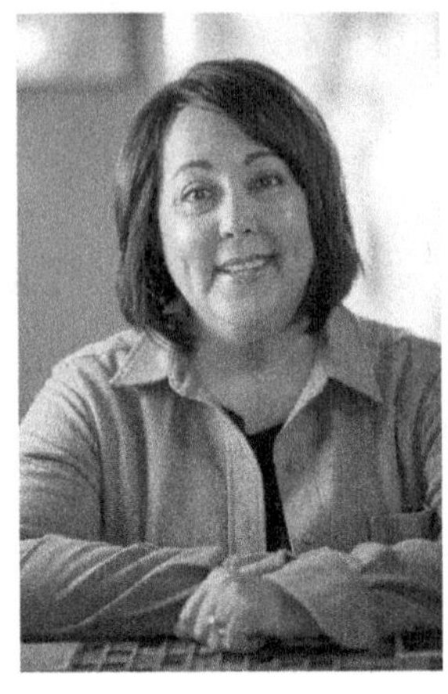 Kim Blaufuss is a practicing Chinese Medical Provider and Acupuncturist. She lives in the Pacific Northwest with her husband, two horses, and four cats. Her practice and writing focus on using Chinese Medicine every day to balance emotions and embrace the past.

In her first book on the topic, Kim introduces you to her love of Five Element Theory. Based on her own experience as a caregiver for her mother and sister, Kim shares how she incorporated her background in Chinese Medicine to help her navigate the turmoil that can arise in caregiving.

To learn more, check out her practice at best-acupuncture.com or her Youtube @bestacupuncturellc.